Diabetes Cookbook & Meal Plan for the Newly Diagnosed

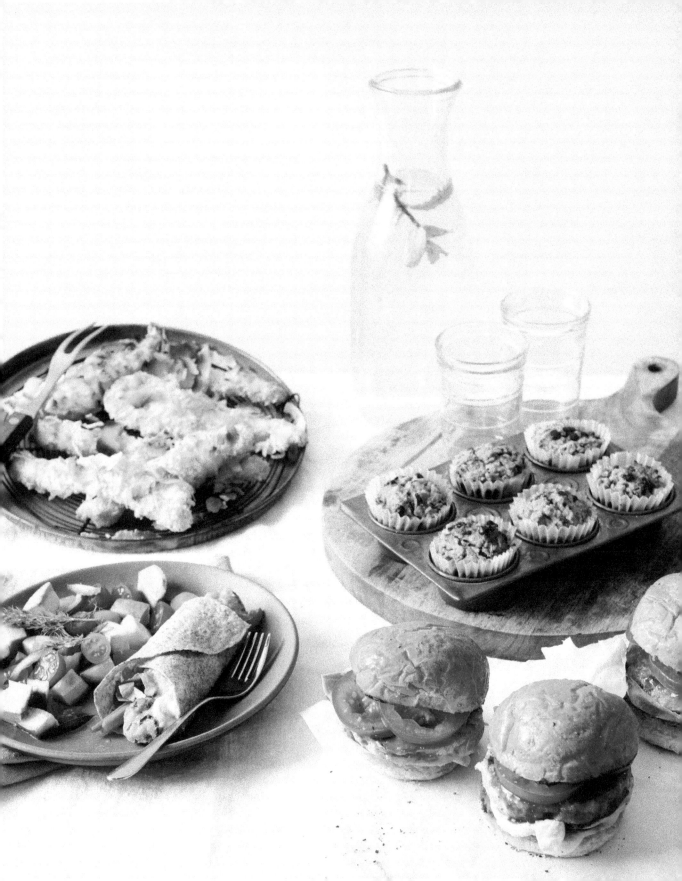

Diabetes Cookbook & Meal Plan

for the
NEWLY DIAGNOSED

Lori Zanini, RD, CDE

Photography by
MARIJA VIDAL

ROCKRIDGE
PRESS

ISBN: Print 978-1-64152-023-2
eBook 978-1-64152-024-9

To my husband, Grant, and my son, Preston.
Thank you both for your endless love & support,
and for being constant sources of motivation.

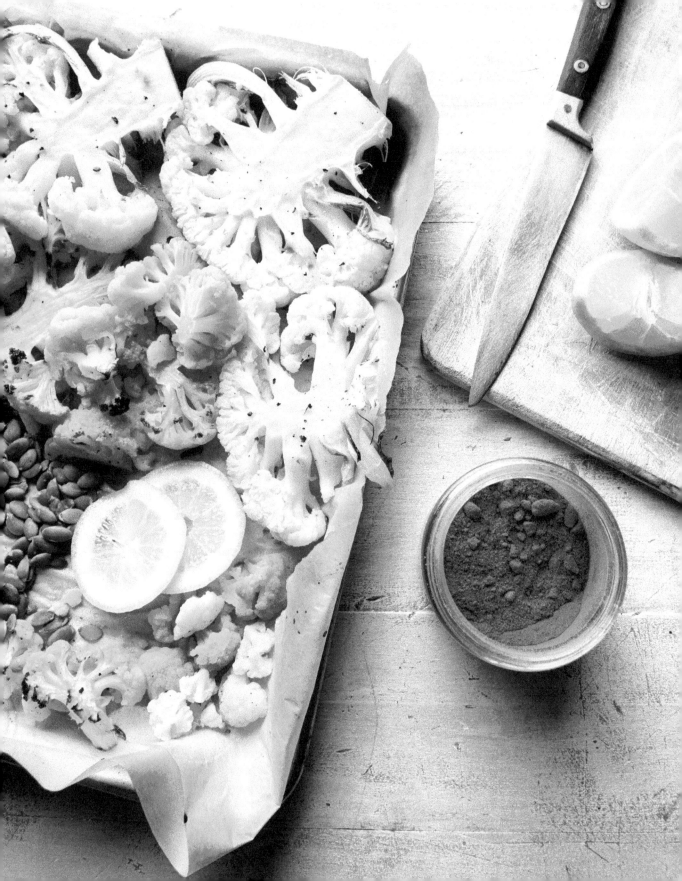

Contents

Introduction

If you have recently been diagnosed with type 2 diabetes and are feeling confused, overwhelmed, and not exactly sure where to start, you are in the right place. Having worked as a registered dietitian and diabetes educator for more than 10 years, I've heard firsthand the frustrations and fears that a diabetes diagnosis can bring. I've listened as clients expressed their anger, disappointment, and sadness. And most importantly, I've given them the tools to empower themselves when they express the desire to change.

While getting a diagnosis of type 2 is no simple matter, please know that you can both manage and control diabetes so that you never have to worry about the negative side effects it could potentially have on your life and health.

The best time to take action is now, when you are newly diagnosed, because you still have time to prevent diabetes-related complications and bring your blood sugar back down to normal (yes, normal) levels. I'll give you everything you need to understand how food affects your blood sugar and exactly what you can do to control it—today. Here are some of the helpful and life-changing tools you will find in this book.

- Four weeks of expertly designed meal plans. These meal plans are both customizable and easy to follow, so they are sure to meet both your nutritional and lifestyle needs.

- More than 100 quick and easy, balanced recipes that taste delicious and have wholesome and nourishing ingredients your entire family will love. There is truly something for everyone.

- My popular Complete the Plate method to balanced eating. Continuing from my first cookbook, this simple graphic, presented alongside each recipe, will give you insight into how to mix and match recipes to create complete meals.

- Education so you can understand exactly what a type 2 diabetes diagnosis is and what it means for you. We'll discuss what's within your control (spoiler alert: There's a lot!) and how food and lifestyle factors can greatly benefit you.

- Science-backed solutions and answers to common questions. Is diabetes reversible? What is the difference between prediabetes, type 1 diabetes, and type 2 diabetes? What specific concerns should I discuss with my doctor? Are there any mental health considerations I need to know about? What about medications? All of these questions and more will be addressed.

- Practical advice for managing diabetes in the real world. Topics include what to order in your favorite restaurants, how to navigate special occasions, stress-free planning and preparing of meals, how to

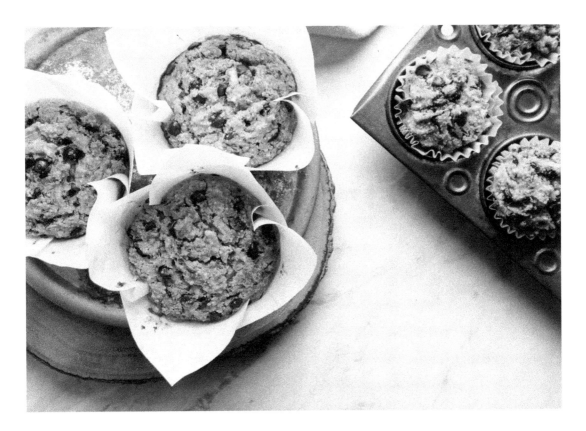

enjoy social events, what to do when you are on the run, and much more!

Growing up in the South (hey, Nashville!), I learned from a very young age that food should be both nourishing *and* delicious. And if you read my first book, *Eat What You Love Diabetes Cookbook*, you already know that I wholeheartedly believe everyone should enjoy and savor their food, and it's quite possible to do this *while* improving your health. As a registered dietitian, I firmly attest to the power of food, especially when it comes to managing type 2 diabetes. And you don't have to give up flavor when you are putting your health

first. In developing the recipes for this book, I focused on flavor, variety, comfort, and consistency. These meals should be seen as tasty solutions rather than bland inconveniences.

This book will equip you with the confidence and information you need to thrive with diabetes for the rest of your life. You will learn how to take control of the decisions you make every day while being empowered with the resources to know what's best for your body. Research has proven that early intervention improves long-term health outcomes when it comes to type 2 diabetes, so congratulations on starting your journey!

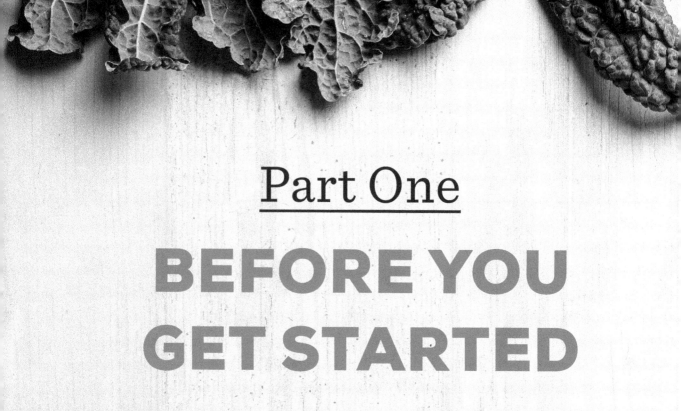

Part One

BEFORE YOU GET STARTED

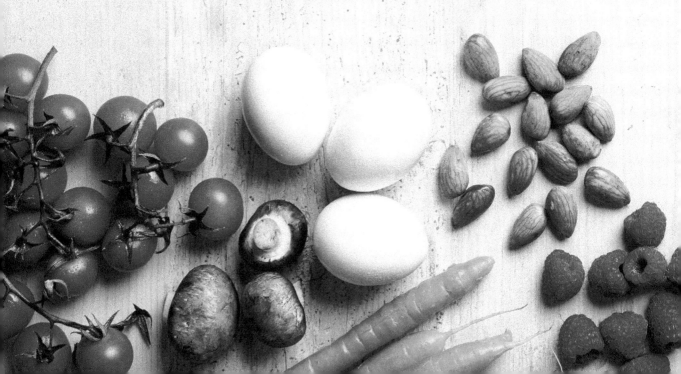

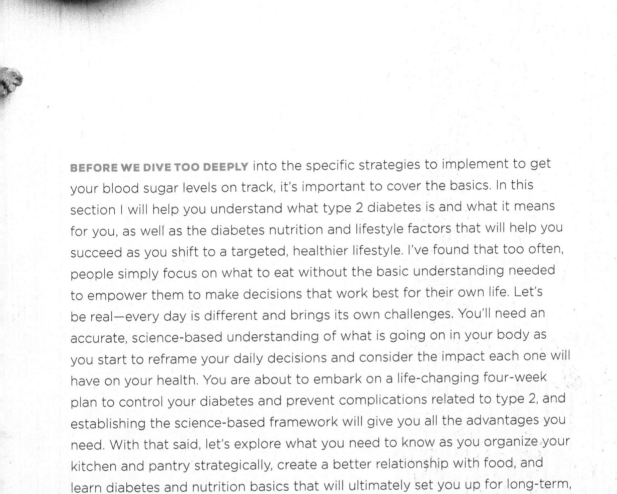

BEFORE WE DIVE TOO DEEPLY into the specific strategies to implement to get your blood sugar levels on track, it's important to cover the basics. In this section I will help you understand what type 2 diabetes is and what it means for you, as well as the diabetes nutrition and lifestyle factors that will help you succeed as you shift to a targeted, healthier lifestyle. I've found that too often, people simply focus on what to eat without the basic understanding needed to empower them to make decisions that work best for their own life. Let's be real—every day is different and brings its own challenges. You'll need an accurate, science-based understanding of what is going on in your body as you start to reframe your daily decisions and consider the impact each one will have on your health. You are about to embark on a life-changing four-week plan to control your diabetes and prevent complications related to type 2, and establishing the science-based framework will give you all the advantages you need. With that said, let's explore what you need to know as you organize your kitchen and pantry strategically, create a better relationship with food, and learn diabetes and nutrition basics that will ultimately set you up for long-term, lasting health and success.

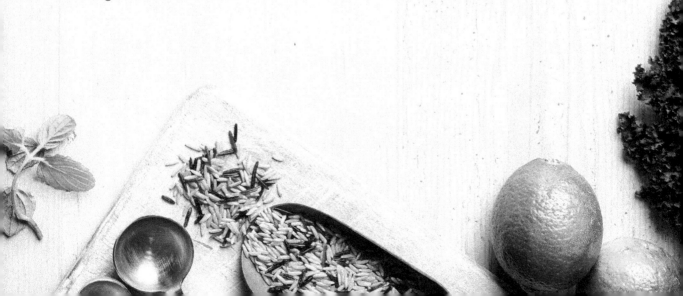

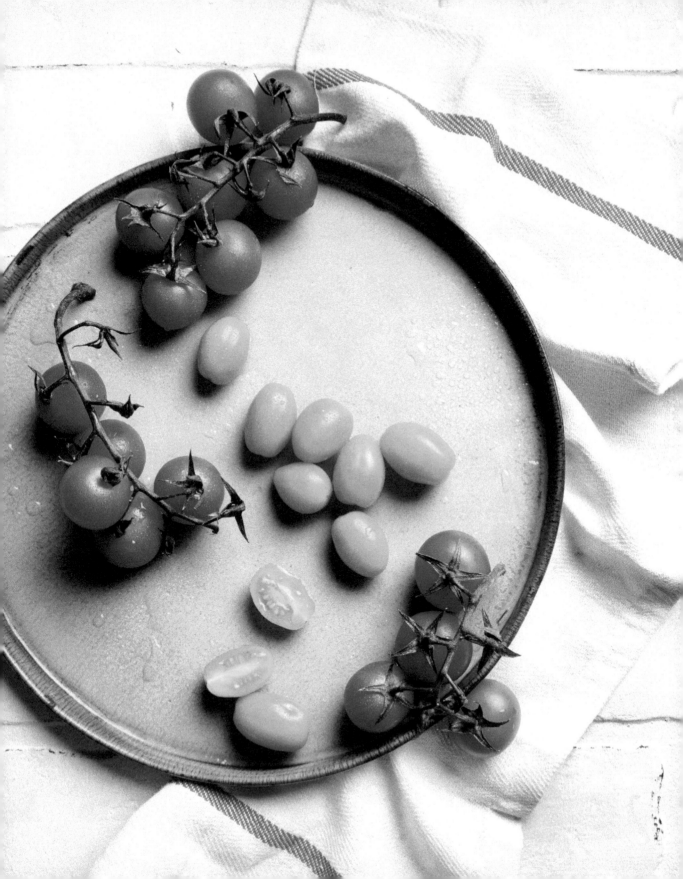

1

Understand What It Means to Be Diagnosed with Type 2

A diabetes diagnosis can undoubtedly be scary, especially when you are first diagnosed. Over the years, I've found that much of the fear comes from the unknown and from stories of complications that can be caused by long periods of time with uncontrolled blood sugar. It is true that people living with uncontrolled diabetes have a higher risk of complications such as heart disease, stroke, vision loss, depression, kidney failure, and other problems. But this doesn't have to be your story.

It's vital to understand that it is absolutely possible for you to control your blood sugar levels and never be a part of any of the scary statistics you may have heard. And it's likely a lot easier than you may think. Well-controlled blood sugar is the goal, as this will prevent any further diabetes-related health problems. In fact, as you begin to follow the nutrition and lifestyle habits you'll learn in this book, it's very likely you will find yourself feeling better than you have in years, and with normal, healthy blood sugar levels.

The diabetes nutrition and lifestyle education strategies you are about to learn will equip you with the tools you need to gain and maintain healthier habits for the rest of your life. Yes, you can change! Plus, you deserve the energy, confidence, and longevity that good health provides. Taking charge of your diabetes will yield immediate results that will continue to propel you forward as you make this a sustainable and enjoyable lifestyle.

Diabetes in America

The current statistics are staggering. According to the latest research from the Centers for Disease Control and Prevention (CDC), 30.3 million American adults are living with diabetes, which translates to almost 10 percent of the entire adult population. And this number is growing by 1.5 million annually. Roughly 90 to 95 percent have type 2 diabetes, making it the most common type of diabetes among American adults, according to the CDC.

While these numbers are certainly shocking, I share them only so that you know you are not alone. These statistics also mean that more programs, resources, and solutions are being created daily to support an underserved population. Why? Because we need them. Our nation can no longer ignore the need to approach diabetes with research-backed, action-oriented solutions.

As we continue to shed light on the diabetes epidemic and talk about it more often and more openly, we are creating better support for those living with diabetes. It's time to stop feeling ashamed of a diabetes diagnosis,

because it's certainly not your fault. In most cases, the food system, the health care system, and our culture's norms have unwittingly stacked the cards against you.

Rather than feeling overwhelmed or paralyzed with fear, you can now approach a type 2 diabetes diagnosis with a sense of confidence and control, because you can educate and equip yourself with everything you need not only to live but to thrive with diabetes. You have the right and the ability to expect better health outcomes for the rest of your life.

HOW DID WE GET HERE?

As we have progressed as a society, many things have become easier and more efficient. However, with that, we've compromised some important things about our health. As a society, we no longer have to move as much, since cars, computers, and drive-through windows have made everything we need more accessible. And we don't have to cook as often, since fast-food restaurants, processed convenience foods, and time-saving delivery companies have enabled us to always have quick meal options.

Unfortunately, this does not always promote the healthiest of habits. More food options lead many people to diets that are high in calories but offer little nutritional value. This is sometimes referred to as the Standard American Diet—a diet that is low in fiber and high in sugar, salt, unhealthy fats, and other inflammation-causing components.

I encourage my clients to let go of the guilt they may be feeling about the food choices they have made in the past, because it's very likely that the food has failed them! Low-quality ingredients, large portion sizes, and convenience foods are among the key problems that have set us up for failure. The good news is that we have more information and solutions than ever before on what will truly help us lead healthy and active lives. We now know exactly what we should include in our diets to promote long, fulfilling lives. Understanding what's wrong with the Standard American Diet is one of the best ways to set yourself up for future success—just as one single meal can begin to improve your blood sugar levels. Better yet, within a few days, you can be experiencing the results you have been looking for!

Diabetes and the Body

Type 2 diabetes is a metabolic disease, which means it is caused by a problem in the chemical reactions of the body's cells.

In people with type 2 diabetes, the body (specifically, the pancreas) is either not creating enough insulin or not using the insulin properly—a condition called insulin resistance. Insulin resistance will eventually lead to higher-than-normal blood sugar levels. Insulin is the natural hormone that helps you get the sugar from food, known as glucose, into your cells to be used for energy. If the insulin is not used properly (or if you do not have enough), once the carbohydrates you eat are broken down into glucose in your body, this glucose stays in your blood rather than being transported to your cells, where it is supposed to be. This buildup of glucose in the blood is referred to as high blood sugar, or hyperglycemia.

Type 1 diabetes is a different disease, although it also affects insulin production. Type 1 is an autoimmune disease and accounts

Prediabetes and Prevention

In addition to all the people who have been diagnosed with type 2 diabetes, there are an estimated 84 million U.S. adults who have prediabetes—elevated blood sugar. That's more than one out of every three adults! Unfortunately, more than 90 percent of those with prediabetes do not even know they have it. Since a prediabetes diagnosis is often a sign that someone will likely develop type 2 diabetes within the next five years, this is a vital time to implement change.

Prevention is possible, and the first step is awareness. Having your hemoglobin A1c (a three-month average of your blood sugar levels) checked annually will let you know where you stand when it comes to prediabetes and type 2 diabetes. Awareness, diabetes nutrition education, increased physical activity, and a supportive health care team will make all the difference.

for approximately 5 percent of all diabetes cases in the United States. Historically, type 1 diabetes has been referred to as juvenile diabetes because the average age of diagnosis is approximately 14. Individuals living with type 1 diabetes require insulin therapy because their pancreas does not make any insulin at all. It is not the case that anyone who is taking insulin has type 1 diabetes. I like to point out that using insulin to manage blood sugar levels, in people with type 1 or type 2 diabetes, does not mean they have poor blood sugar control. In fact, insulin is one of the most natural ways to manage blood sugar levels (if medicine is needed), since that is what our bodies naturally make to regulate blood sugar.

Symptoms of the onset of type 2 diabetes can vary from one person to the next. High blood sugar levels can often cause slow healing of cuts, fatigue, frequent urination, increased thirst, headaches, blurred vision, unintended weight loss—and sometimes there are no symptoms at all. If you experience any of these symptoms, it's always best to notify your health care team and check your blood sugar levels.

It's important to mention that type 2 diabetes is a chronic disease, meaning it is long-lasting. However, it's also vital to note that type 2 diabetes is different from most other chronic diseases because it can be self-managed. What you do every day will have a huge impact on your long-term health. While type 2 diabetes cannot be cured, it can be managed and go into remission. You can have diabetes *and* normal, controlled blood sugar levels, which is the ultimate goal that will provide the best quality of life and prevent any future complications related to diabetes.

Questions Your Doctor Wishes You Would Ask

CAN I EXERCISE? If so, do I have any limitations? I've often called physical movement and activity "free medicine," because it is a powerful way to improve blood sugar levels right away. Be sure to get specific guidance and clearance from your doctor before you start moving. YouTube videos, water aerobics, outdoor hikes, Zumba, stretching, yoga, and strength training can all help. Be sure to pick a form of activity you enjoy, and do it regularly.

WHAT IS MY HEMOGLOBIN A1C? When it comes to a diabetes diagnosis, this is the most important number to know. Your A1c is the average of what your blood sugar level has been throughout the day for the past two to three months. It measures how much sugar is attached to your red blood cells. Knowing this number will give you the big picture of how well you are controlling your diabetes.

HERE ARE THE RANGES:
- Normal: Less than 5.7 percent
- Borderline (also called prediabetes): 5.7 to 6.4 percent
- Diabetes: 6.5 percent or greater

Once someone has been diagnosed with type 2 diabetes, the aim is to keep hemoglobin A1c below 7 percent. You always want to check with your doctor to see if he or she has specific and personal goals for you, but these are the general guidelines from the American Diabetes Association.

HOW DO MY MEDICATIONS WORK? When should I take them? What should I do if I forget a dose? If you have been given any medications to help with your blood sugar levels, it's important to understand the why *and* the how. Ask your doctor to explain why he or she is choosing the particular medication and how you should take it. Make sure it is a medication you are able to afford every day. The more you know about your medications, the better you will be able to take them and recognize how well they are working or report any unusual side effects.

CAN I HAVE A BLOOD SUGAR MONITOR? Checking blood sugar levels at home is one of the best ways to immediately understand how food, exercise, sleep, and other lifestyle habits affect your blood sugar daily. Ask your doctor when you should check your blood sugar level and what your goal levels should be.

You can check your blood sugar levels at any time you like throughout the day. However, it's especially helpful to check your fasting or premeal blood sugar level and check again two hours after the first bite of your meal to accurately determine how the food is affecting your blood sugar. The American Diabetes Association recommends that fasting or premeal blood sugar level be between 70 and 130 mg/dL; two hours after the first bite of a meal, it should be less than 180 mg/dL.

Diabetes and Common Treatments

If you have been newly diagnosed with diabetes, you may be wondering what treatments are available to you. Let's review the most common ways of treating this disease.

DIET

Seeking nutrition education from a nutrition expert has been found to be highly effective. Registered dietitians who are also certified diabetes educators are the best source of science-based, credible diabetes nutrition education. They are able to provide medical nutrition therapy (MNT), which is a diet specifically created and customized for those with diabetes. Research has found that MNT from a registered dietitian can help lower hemoglobin A1c for people with type 2 diabetes by 0.3 to 2.0 percent, according to the American Diabetes Association.

It's important to realize there isn't only one way to success when modifying what you eat to manage diabetes. Several different meal-planning strategies and methods have been found to work. Of those that have been most studied, the Mediterranean diet, the DASH diet, and vegetarian and plant-based foods have all been shown to be helpful in both preventing diabetes and managing it.

PHYSICAL ACTIVITY

Physical activity encompasses many different types of movement and is critical to include in all diabetes management plans. Participating in a structured exercise plan for at least eight consecutive weeks has been found to reduce hemoglobin A1c levels by up to 0.66 percent, even if there is no change in weight, according to research published in 2001 in the *Journal of the American Medical Association*. This is quite significant and should be a big motivation to get you moving. As you lose weight, your A1c should go down even more.

The goal is for adults with type 2 diabetes to engage in 150 minutes of physical activity each week, spread over at least three days a week. To experience the most benefits, it's also recommended to go no more than two consecutive days without exercising.

While this physical activity recommendation can seem daunting if you are not currently doing much exercise, be encouraged that it's completely fine to start where you are and continue to increase the intensity and duration as you are able. Flexibility, strength, and balance training are also helpful.

MEDICATION

Depending on your individual situation, your health care provider may recommend medication. Please don't view a medication prescription as a failure. Over the years as I have taught diabetes education, I've had patients compare their personal situations—some were on no medications, some were on insulin, some were on multiple oral medications—and judge themselves based on this comparison.

It is a myth that people who are not taking any medications at all have better blood sugar numbers than those who do take medications. At the end of the day there is one goal: To keep your blood sugar levels as well controlled as possible, because that is the number one way to prevent complications related to diabetes. Taking diabetes medications does not mean you will always have to be on them, nor does it mean you have failed in your efforts to control your blood sugar. It means at that moment, your health care team believes you need them. It is important to ask questions about how to take your medication properly and to be sure to do so.

INSULIN THERAPY

Insulin is actually one of the most natural ways to lower blood sugar levels, since this is what your body naturally produces to keep your blood sugar levels controlled. For this reason, I always encourage my clients to not be worried about starting insulin therapy. It does not mean you have failed. In fact, it is estimated that up to 50 percent of individuals with diabetes will require insulin within 10 years of their diagnosis, according to the UK Prospective Diabetes Study.

While every person is different, it is generally accepted that an individual can take up to three oral diabetes medications before being switched to insulin. There are two main types of insulin, basal (long acting) and bolus (short acting). Bolus insulin is taken before a meal to help lower postmeal blood sugar, so knowing how many carbohydrates you will be eating is especially important when taking bolus insulin. Examples of bolus insulin that you may have heard of include glulisine (Apidra), aspart (NovoLog), and lispro (Humalog). These types of insulin can start working within 5 to 15 minutes and will last less than five hours.

Basal insulin works to control blood sugar levels between meals and throughout the evening. Common examples of basal insulin are detemir (Levemir) and glargine (Lantus). Detemir will start working within three to eight hours, and glargine within two to four hours. Both can last up to 24 hours, so you can see the value of taking basal insulin.

There are also combinations of insulin available as well as new medications and types of insulin that are being approved by the Food and Drug Administration (FDA) literally every month. Your personal pharmacist can be an invaluable resource about these types of insulin and medications, so try to have all of your medications and/or insulin filled at the same pharmacy to add an extra pair of expert eyes.

While there is no cure for diabetes, you absolutely can manage and control it by paying attention to what you eat, increasing your physical activity, maintaining a healthy weight, and taking medication, if necessary. Know your options and make the best plan for yourself with your health care team.

Diabetes and Mental Health

It is very common for a type 2 diabetes diagnosis to cause a wide range of emotions. If the changes needed to control your blood sugar levels are leaving you feeling overwhelmed and stressed, you are certainly not alone. Please know this is normal and expected. During this time, it's essential to pay attention to and acknowledge how you are feeling, enlist support, and practice good self-care.

A study recently published in *Current Diabetes Reports* found that people living with diabetes may have twice the risk of depression. In addition, fluctuations in blood sugar levels can mimic symptoms of anxiety and depression. When your blood sugar is too high, it can cause fatigue and trouble concentrating, while low blood sugar can cause feelings of nervousness and anxiety.

Clearly, you need to make sure you are taking a holistic approach to your health and focusing on your entire well-being, including your mental health. I encourage you to speak with your physician about any concerns you may have and to consider adding a mental health professional to your diabetes health care team.

Support and Diabetes

Help can come in many forms. Understand the options that are available to you.

- **Your health care team (primary care physician, endocrinologist, certified diabetes educator, registered dietitian, nurse, etc.):** These clinicians can simplify your daily diabetes plan to make it easier to follow.
- **Trained mental health professionals (marriage and family therapist, licensed clinical social worker, etc.):** These individuals are trained to be the caring, supportive professionals you need during difficult times.
- **Telehealth:** Many insurance companies now provide access to professionals over the phone. Check with your particular insurance plan to see if anything is available to you. Many times it is free or there is only a copay.
- **Local support groups:** There is so much power in being with others who are going through exactly what you are. Check your local hospitals, medical groups, and other health programs to see what may be available.

- **Yoga and movement classes:** Starting gentle programs will help ease stress levels and provide a new opportunity to meet others.
- **Online education:** Ongoing education is important to provide solutions that will help prevent burnout and ease stress levels. Identify reputable websites by whether they quote research studies and have qualified professionals writing the content or being quoted as the experts. I also offer a step-by-step diabetes management program at www.fortheloveofdiabetes.com.
- **Online support:** This can come in many forms. Some of my favorite reputable organizations that offer online support are the American Diabetes Association, Diabetes Sisters, and various Facebook groups.

Is Type 2 Diabetes Reversible?

Whether or not type 2 diabetes can be reversed is one of the most common questions I am asked. While some studies, such as a 2013 study published in *Diabetes Care*, have found that diabetes can be reversed, it is often by extreme weight loss measures such as bariatric surgery or very-low-calorie diets (800 calories or less per day). As expected, other side effects and complications, such as vitamin deficiencies and mental health concerns, can arise secondary to these drastic changes.

The most important aspect of controlling diabetes is long-term blood sugar control. It is possible to be diagnosed with type 2 diabetes yet maintain normal blood sugar levels throughout the day, and this is the goal. Remember that normal blood sugar levels can be achieved through diet and lifestyle changes.

While it is never too late to change, newly diagnosed individuals have a greater chance of normalizing their blood sugar levels when they change their habits soon after their initial type 2 diabetes diagnosis.

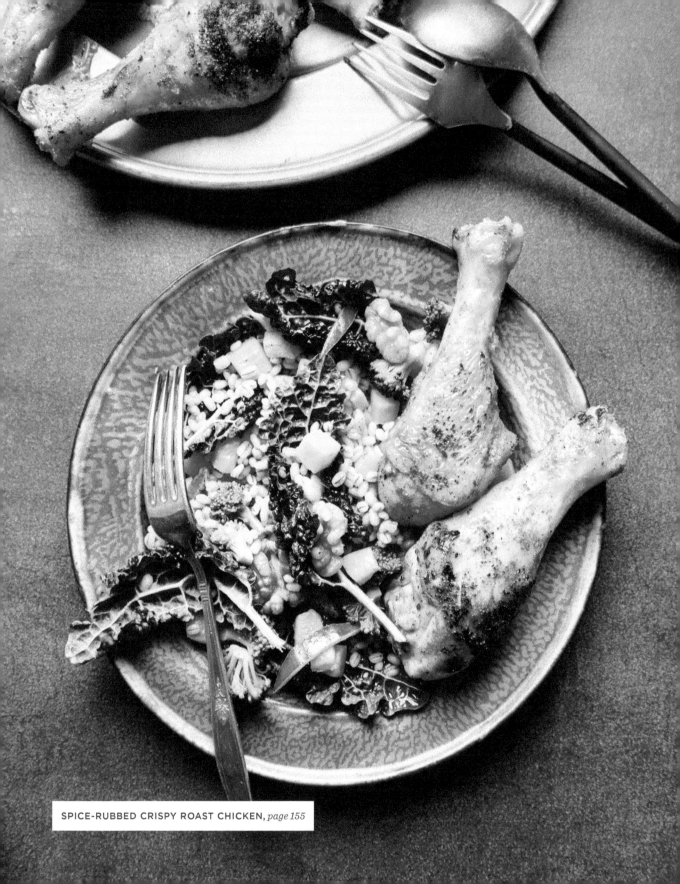

SPICE-RUBBED CRISPY ROAST CHICKEN, *page 155*

2

Get Educated about Diabetes Nutrition

Understanding what is in your food and how it can affect your blood sugar levels can seem like a daunting task. But it's important to first learn which foods are mostly carbohydrates, mostly protein, and mostly fat so you can learn the best foods to choose, the appropriate amounts, and the best times to eat them. Having a good grasp of diabetes nutrition basics will help you make the best decisions in any setting—and you will be surprised to discover that it's a lot less complicated than it may seem.

Food is one of the oldest forms of medicine, and that is especially true when it comes to living with diabetes. Taking control of what you eat will have immediate benefits to your health. As mentioned in the previous chapter, research has shown that MNT provided by a registered dietitian can decrease hemoglobin A1c levels by up to 2 percent, so it's definitely worth the effort to learn about and implement the strategies in this chapter and to seek additional help as needed.

Nutrients and the Newly Diagnosed

You do not need to follow one specific eating plan to be successful. In fact, research has shown that there are many different nutrition plans that can help you manage your diabetes. What is important is to learn some key principles that you can implement in a way that works for you. Individualizing your plan to meet your budget, food preferences, scheduling demands, and family needs will make all the difference.

I focus on what to *include* in your meals, rather than simply what to avoid, and I hope you will find my approach refreshing. Too often, diets teach us to restrict certain foods entirely, leaving us with more questions than answers. When we are told that we can't eat something, we end up craving those off-limits foods more than we would otherwise. There is a better way.

This chapter will give you a deeper look at exactly what foods to add to your daily meals and teach you why they are important, so you will be empowered to make better choices in any situation you may find yourself.

At the end of the day, eating well with diabetes is simply following a healthy nutrition plan—one than anyone could benefit from eating. So please don't be discouraged and feel as if you need to eat completely differently than everyone else around you. You can and should enjoy your food! So with that, let's dive a little deeper.

MACRONUTRIENTS

Macronutrients are essential nutrients the body requires for growth, metabolism, and other vital functions. They provide energy in the form of calories and are classified into three main groups: Carbohydrates, protein, and fat. Let's take a closer look at each.

CARBOHYDRATES

Perhaps the nutrient most perceived as a villain, carbohydrates often get an unnecessarily bad rap. But let's be clear, you do not have to completely eliminate or avoid carbohydrates to control your blood sugar levels. In fact, carbohydrates are an important energy source that helps your cells function optimally. What you have to pay attention to is the type of carbohydrates you choose and how much of them you eat.

Starches, sugars, and fiber are all considered carbohydrates (aka carbs). Starches and fiber are complex carbs, meaning they are made of long chains of multiple sugar molecules. Sugars are simple carbs, which means your body will digest them more quickly, so they have the potential to raise your blood sugar levels faster than starches and fiber.

Some simple carbohydrates are very healthy and beneficial to your overall health, so they do not need to be omitted from your eating plans. Examples include full-fat dairy products and fruit. The latest research points to the benefits of choosing organic, grass-fed, full-fat dairy products, such as kefir, yogurt, and whole milk, for people with type 2 diabetes. You do not need to eliminate fruit, but do be mindful of the amount and frequency in your meals. As a general rule, I tell my clients to make sure they are eating more vegetables than fruits throughout the day and to choose the highest-fiber fruits, like berries, most often.

It's important to note that most of the simple carbs in a typical American diet are added to foods, often without our being aware of them, so it's important to read labels for added sugar, like high-fructose corn syrup, fruit juice concentrate, brown sugar, and cane sugar. These types of added sugars are digested within five minutes and quickly raise blood sugar levels. One of the best health decisions anyone can make is to commit to identifying and eliminating as much added sugar as possible, to avoid the multitude of complications it can create.

Complex carbohydrates are best for blood sugar control because they are higher in fiber, are digested more slowly (taking up to 90 minutes), and contain more nutrients. Since they are digested more slowly, they will also keep you satisfied for longer compared with simple sugars.

Starches are what people typically think of when they say "carbs." These include cereals, breads, pastas, peas, bagels, and rice. While you can still eat these foods, you should limit the portion size and the frequency, and choose whole-grain options. If you choose refined white starches, they will offer little nutritional value, be digested quickly, and subsequently raise your blood sugar levels. Additionally, they won't keep you full for very long, so while they have the same number of calories per gram as protein (4 calories per gram), it's easy to overeat them.

It's important to include adequate amounts of fiber in your diet every day, and you may find that challenging. The goal is 25 grams per day for women and 38 grams per day for men. Fiber occurs naturally in the cell walls of plant foods, so including more vegetables, whole grains, beans, nuts, seeds, and high-fiber fruits (such as berries and apples) will ensure better health.

Quick recap: Dairy products, fruit, whole grains, beans, starchy vegetables (such as potatoes, peas, winter squash, and corn), and added sugar in all its forms all contain carbohydrates. Limit the simple sugars, check labels for added sugars, and start to notice how big your portion sizes of carbohydrates are. (Later in this chapter I'll talk about how carbs fit into the whole diet, servings, and the Complete the Plate method.)

PROTEIN

Protein is also considered an energy nutrient—like carbs, it provides energy in the form of calories. Almost everything in your body requires protein, and protein is found in every cell in your body. Protein supplies the same number of calories per gram as carbohydrates (4 calories), but it takes a lot longer to digest (around two or three hours). This is an important difference, because eating protein with carbohydrates can help stabilize blood sugar levels, since protein does not affect blood sugar levels as much as carbohydrates. For this reason, I recommend including a protein-rich food every time you eat. A study published in 2015 in *Diabetes Care* showed that the order in which we eat foods can be helpful, so eating a protein before a carbohydrate in the same meal may have even better blood sugar results.

When it comes to protein, there are two primary categories: animal-based and plant-based. Examples of healthy animal-based protein include fish, poultry, grass-fed red meats, pork tenderloin, eggs, and cheese. Healthy plant-based protein includes nuts, seeds, beans, tofu, lentils, nut and seed butters, and quinoa. Remember that plant-based foods, which include plant protein, also contain fiber, while animal protein does not, so you can see that including plant-based protein more often in your diet will give you the best results. It's also important to note that plant-based protein is easier on the kidneys than animal-based protein.

Studies, including a study published in 2017 in the *Journal of Geriatric Cardiology*, have found that ensuring you are primarily eating plant-based foods, including plant-based protein, is highly beneficial for treating type 2 diabetes. This does not mean you need to become vegan or vegetarian; it simply means you should aim to eat more plant protein than animal protein overall. We live in a society that has access to cheap, low-quality protein sources (think Quarter Pounders with Cheese), so most of us are eating enough protein; it's the quality and type of protein that will make all the difference.

FAT

The final type of macronutrient that supplies energy is fat. Fat takes longer to digest than carbohydrates or protein, so it will help keep you satisfied for hours after meals. Fat helps your immune system function properly, helps your body absorb certain vitamins A, D, E, and K efficiently; provides structure for cell membranes; and regulates body temperature. As you can see, fat is an essential component of your diet. Fat provides a more concentrated fuel source, having 9 calories per gram. As with the other macronutrients, it's all about the amount and type of fat that you are consuming.

Fat is either saturated or unsaturated, having to do with its chemical structure. Saturated fats are solid at room temperature, and unsaturated fats are liquid at room temperature. The unsaturated fats are further broken down into polyunsaturated and monounsaturated fats, again having to do with their chemical structure.

When it comes to the type of fat you are consuming, unsaturated fats are the best. Examples of foods that contain monounsaturated fats include olive oil, avocados, nuts, and nut butters. (Pro tip: Look for nut butters that have oil on the top; this is actually a sign that it's a better choice.)

Polyunsaturated fats are essential fats, meaning your body can't produce them, so you must get them from food. The best types of polyunsaturated fats are omega-3 fatty acids, because they have been shown to have powerful benefits in reducing the risk of heart disease and stroke. Examples of foods that contain omega-3 fatty acids include salmon, sardines, ground flaxseed, walnuts, mackerel, oysters, halibut, and fresh tuna.

Saturated fats have been the subject of much debate and recently have become more accepted than in previous years as the science of nutrition has advanced. However, they should still be consumed in moderate amounts, and their health benefits do not outweigh those of omega-3 fats and monounsaturated fats. Examples include coconut oil, ghee, butter, whole dairy products, and meat.

The most harmful type of fat is a type of saturated fat called trans fat. It is created when a manufacturer adds an extra hydrogen molecule to a saturated fat in a process called hydrogenation. Trans fat offers no dietary benefits and should be completely eliminated. Trans fat will both raise your LDL (bad) cholesterol and lower your HDL (good) cholesterol, thus damaging your heart health in multiple ways. Check food ingredient lists and avoid anything that has the word hydrogenated. Examples of foods that could potentially have trans fats include coffee creamer; peanut butter made with hydrogenated oil; commercially prepared cookies, cakes, and crackers; biscuits; and stick margarines.

Again, fat is a necessary macronutrient that your body requires, and it's a good idea to include a healthy source of fat every time you eat. The ultimate goal is to eliminate all trans fat and switch to mostly monounsaturated and omega-3 fats.

Using all of this information about macronutrients, I like to point out to my clients that eating something with quickly digested, refined carbs combined with a high-fat food will likely keep blood sugar

Rethinking Fat and Cholesterol

You may notice that cholesterol and saturated fat content are not listed among the nutrition facts for the recipes in this book. This is because the latest research published in the *American Journal of Clinical Nutrition* shows that the cholesterol we eat in food is not the leading contributor to blood cholesterol levels, and there is no conclusive evidence that eating cholesterol and saturated fat increases the risk of heart disease. In fact, the 2015–2020 Dietary Guidelines for Americans (which you can find at www.choosemyplate.gov/dietary-guidelines) removed the previous recommendation to limit cholesterol intake to 300 milligrams per day, stating that adequate evidence was simply not available for that recommendation. Rather, lifestyle factors, such as obesity, physical inactivity, and a diet high in sugar and processed carbohydrates seem to play a larger role in cardiovascular disease risk, according to the American Heart Association and research published in *JAMA Internal Medicine*. Nevertheless, limiting your overall intake of foods high in saturated fat (which all of the recipes in this book do) is still part of a healthy way of eating, and having balance in the diet is key to properly nourishing the body.

levels elevated for longer periods of time. Examples of this type of meal include traditional pepperoni pizza, meat lasagna, and macaroni and cheese. Each of these foods can be made healthier and create less of a blood sugar spike, though. For example, thin-crust whole-wheat veggie pizza, vegetarian lasagna made with zucchini instead of pasta, and macaroni and cheese made with whole-wheat macaroni and with veggies added are all better alternatives.

OTHER ESSENTIAL NUTRIENTS

In addition to the macronutrients, there are other vitamins, minerals, and nutrients that play key roles in managing type 2 diabetes. It's helpful to know what they are and where they can be found so you can make sure you are getting the right amount in your own diet.

VITAMIN D

Vitamin D is important for everyone but especially for those with type 2 diabetes. Vitamin D is used in nearly every part of the body. It plays a role in your immune system, assists with the absorption of calcium, and helps regulate cell growth.

Historically, we received "the sunshine vitamin" from more frequent exposure to the outdoors, but with jobs being primarily indoors these days, most of us simply aren't getting enough of this vital vitamin. Since vitamin D deficiency can lead to decreased insulin secretion, which will subsequently increase blood sugar levels, it's necessary to make sure people with type 2 diabetes are getting enough, and supplements may be necessary, according to a 2011 study in *Diabetes Spectrum*.

FOOD	VITAMIN D (IU)
Swordfish, cooked (3 ounces)	566
Salmon, cooked (3 ounces)	447
Vitamin D-fortified milk (1 cup)	115
2 sardines (packed in oil, drained)	46
Egg (1 large)	41
Light tuna, packed in water, drained (3 ounces)	40
Shiitake mushrooms (½ cup)	25

References: National Institutes of Health, "Vitamin D Fact Sheet for Health Professionals"; American Dietetic Association, "Complete Food and Nutrition Guide"

The Recommended Dietary Allowance (RDA) of vitamin D for individuals 9 to 70 years of age is 600 International Units (IU) per day, according to the FDA. For those older than 70, the recommendation increases to 800 IU per day. Unfortunately, it is difficult to get enough vitamin D from the food we eat. There are a few good sources listed in the chart on the previous page.

I encourage you to be proactive and ask to have your vitamin D levels checked by your health care provider to see where you stand. Discuss whether you need a supplement and what you can do to ensure you are getting enough vitamin D every day.

MAGNESIUM

Magnesium is a mineral found in many foods including leafy green vegetables, nuts, seeds, legumes, avocados, and whole grains. It is extremely helpful since it plays a role in regulating blood pressure, supporting muscle and nerve function, producing neurotransmitters, maintaining strong bones, forming proteins, and producing energy through the breakdown of glucose in the body. So yes, it's *really* important!

The RDA for magnesium is 400 to 420 milligrams per day for men and 310 to 320 milligrams per day for women, and fewer than 60 percent of American adults are getting enough. New research from multiple scientific studies has uncovered the role magnesium plays in preventing type 2 diabetes. In fact, a recent analysis published in the *Journal of Internal Medicine* found that the risk of developing diabetes was reduced by 15 percent for every 100-milligram-per-day increase in total magnesium intake.

The good news is that it's very easy to add more magnesium to your diet. Getting enough magnesium will help regulate the amount of insulin produced by the pancreas, which helps reduce insulin resistance.

While there is not yet enough evidence to prove that increasing magnesium intake will lower blood glucose levels in people already diagnosed with diabetes, there *is* evidence that people with uncontrolled diabetes tend to have low magnesium levels in their blood due to high blood sugar, causing more magnesium to be lost in the urine, according to the National Institutes of Health. This magnesium deficiency might impair insulin production, which can worsen diabetes control.

A quick list of high-magnesium foods that are also diabetes-friendly is on page 18.

FOOD	MAGNESIUM (MG)
Almonds, dry roasted (1 ounce)	80
Spinach, cooked (½ cup)	78
Cashews, roasted (1 ounce)	74
Peanuts, roasted (¼ cup)	63
Organic soymilk (1 cup)	61
Black beans, cooked (½ cup)	60
Quinoa, cooked (½ cup)	59
Edamame, shelled (½ cup)	50
Natural peanut butter, smooth (2 tablespoons)	49
Avocado, cubed (1 cup)	44
Plain low-fat yogurt (8 ounces)	42
Whole-wheat bread (1 slice)	37
Oatmeal, cooked (½ cup)	32
Halibut, cooked (3 ounces)	24
Chicken breast, roasted (3 ounces)	22
Light tuna, packed in water, drained (3 ounces)	20

SODIUM

It's no secret that there is an excessive amount of sodium, which comes from salt, in the American diet. I often tell my clients that if their food came in a box, bag, or can or through a window, it likely contains too much sodium. The majority of the sodium that gets into your diet comes from foods you eat outside of the home. When you eat fresh, whole foods and cook your meals at home, the sodium levels will significantly decrease (as long as you aren't adding a lot of salt to your food at home, of course). Evidence supports aiming for 1,500 to 2,300 milligrams of sodium per day. To put this into perspective, 1 teaspoon of table salt contains 2,300 milligrams of sodium.

According to the CDC, around 90 percent of Americans ages two and up eat too much sodium on a daily basis—the average daily intake of sodium is over 3,400 milligrams. Excess salt can increase fluid retention, which can force your kidneys to work harder, increase blood pressure, and put you at a greater risk of cardiovascular disease.

Looking at food labels, adding less salt to your meals, and cooking more at home will all help you keep your daily sodium levels in check.

What a Healthy Eating Plan for Type 2 Diabetes Looks Like

In this section we are going to explore some of the most common misconceptions when it comes to what to eat to control your blood sugar after a type 2 diabetes diagnosis. Learning how

to look at your eating plan as a whole, rather than simply what foods you should or shouldn't eat, will help manage your expectations and clarify what you need to do to stay healthy.

In the long run, your overall eating patterns are much more important than any single food or even a single meal. Additionally, setting realistic and achievable goals in the beginning as to what needs to change and how to change it will get you on the fast track to success.

THE WHOLE DIET FOR PEOPLE WITH DIABETES

Often when I meet with clients for the first time, they are excited to report, "I've already stopped eating all carbs!" However, when we talk about this more, it usually means they have stopped eating refined starches such as white bread, pasta, rice, bagels, and donuts. When I ask if they are still eating beans, fruit, and yogurt (just to name a few carb-heavy foods), they usually reply that they are.

While this is a good start, I am much more interested in what you *are* eating than what you are avoiding, because avoidance alone doesn't necessarily make you healthy. A vegetarian diet can include cheese pizza and potato chips, and a gluten-free diet can include a daily steak—you can see where I'm going.

As you start to improve your eating habits, look at what you can *add* to your meals that will increase the nourishing and disease-fighting vitamins, minerals, and nutrients needed to combat type 2 diabetes. Know that blood sugar isn't the only concern. Having type 2 diabetes can also make it more challenging to control blood pressure

Complete the Plate

Full Plate

¼ Plate (Protein)

¼ Plate (Starch)

½ Plate (Protein + Starch)

¾ Plate (Veg + Starch)

¾ Plate (Veg + Protein)

½ Plate (Veg)

½ Plate Nonstarchy Vegetables

¼ Plate Healthy Protein

¼ Plate Carbs

and cholesterol levels, so you need to keep in mind sodium content, healthy fat portions, and maintaining adequate hydration.

The whole-diet approach will help you focus on nutrients rather than merely calories or carbohydrates. Your health and diabetes management are so much more than this! Now, let's dive a little deeper into the specifics.

COMPLETE THE PLATE

One of the easiest ways to succeed any time you eat is to use my Complete the Plate method, a way of looking at meals that I developed. It will give you a quick guide to how balanced your meals are without spending too much time counting carbs.

You will see a color-coded icon with each recipe in this book that will show what portion of the plate the recipe covers. Using a plate that's 9 inches across (it's important, so measure!), the goal is for each meal to contain ½ plate of non-starchy vegetables, ¼ plate of healthy protein, and ¼ plate of high-fiber carbohydrates while including some healthy fats, as well.

If a single recipe in this book does not "complete the plate," you will find suggestions for how best to complete it. These icons will enable you to mix and match various recipes so you can customize your meals to meet your individual preferences and needs.

Nonstarchy vegetables (½ plate): Nonstarchy veggies are high in fiber, antioxidants, and other essential nutrients while being low in carbs and calories. A recent CDC report found that nearly 91 percent of Americans are not eating the recommended 2 to 3 cups per day of vegetables. Making sure they fill half the plate is the first step in building your balanced plate.

Healthy protein (¼ plate): The typical lean protein source contains about 7 grams of protein in every ounce. A good starting point is to aim for 2 to 4 ounces (14 to 28 grams) of protein at every meal and around 1 ounce (7 grams) of protein at snacks. Remember, it's best to choose plant-based protein most often.

High-quality carbohydrates (¼ plate): Remember, you don't need to completely eliminate carbs from your eating plan. Rather, choose the best types in appropriate amounts. Fifteen grams of carbohydrates is 1 serving, and I recommend women have around 30 grams per meal and men around 45 grams of carbs per meal. You may need to adjust this number up or down to meet your personal needs, but this tends to be a good starting point. Snacks should be kept to 15 grams or less and paired with a protein and/or a healthy fat. Below is a list of recommended carbs and the portion sizes for 1 serving (15 grams) of high-quality carbs.

STARCH

- 1 slice 100 percent whole-wheat bread
- ⅓ cup cooked brown rice or whole-wheat pasta
- ½ cup cooked oatmeal
- ½ 100 percent whole-wheat English muffin
- 1 (6-inch) corn or whole-wheat tortilla
- ½ cup green peas
- ½ cup sweet potato
- 1 cup winter squash (butternut, acorn, etc.)
- ½ cup corn
- ⅓ cup cooked quinoa
- ½ cup cooked beans (black, kidney, etc.)
- ½ cup cooked lentils

DAIRY

- 6 ounces plain yogurt
- 6 ounces plain Greek yogurt (contains more protein)
- 8 ounces cow's milk (fat-free or skim milk will raise blood sugar quickly, since it is more liquid, so choose organic full-fat milk)
- 8 ounces unsweetened soy milk (unsweetened almond and coconut milk are very low in carbs)

FRUIT

- ½ grapefruit
- 1 small apple or pear
- 1 cup blackberries or raspberries
- ¾ cup blueberries
- 1⅓ cups strawberries
- 3 dried prunes
- 2 small guavas
- ¾ cup fresh pineapple
- 2 small plums
- 1 small orange
- ⅔ cup pitted cherries

Source: U.S. Department of Agriculture, "Food Composition Databases"

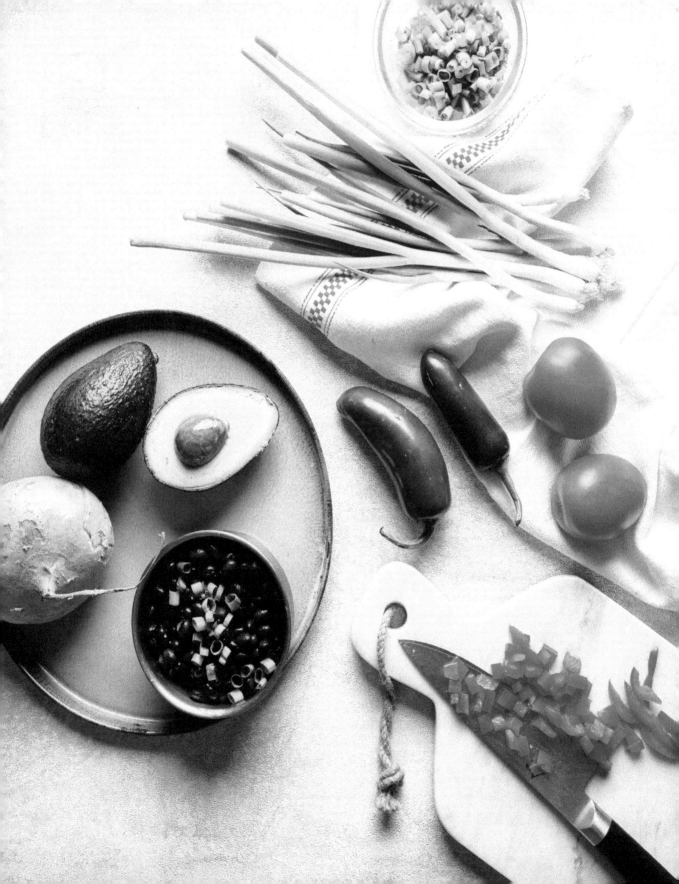

3

Reframe and Rebuild:
Mindful and Practical Planning for the Month Ahead and for Your Lifestyle

As with any change in life, there's more to it than simply knowing what to do. I often tell my clients that while I am an expert in diabetes nutrition, they are the experts in their own lives. They are the ones who will take this information and implement it in a way that works for them. What makes this a truly sustainable lifestyle rather than a temporary diet is the confidence that you will be able to stick to these changes for years to come. Simple, science-based strategies will help propel you forward. Look at this diet and lifestyle change as your launching pad to the long-term habits you will have for the rest of your life.

It's important to be realistic, too. Change isn't always easy. I encourage you to give yourself grace and aim to strive for better, not perfect.

In this chapter we are going to explore some realistic strategies to help you get ready for planning, preparing, and implementing your new eating habits and lifestyle. Know that the attitude you have as you approach this way of eating will make all the difference. These science-based solutions *will* work every single time, and armed with this accurate information and a positive mind-set, you will be sure to succeed!

Reframe Your Thinking

Researchers have found that behavioral change is a process, and it typically takes place over five stages: precontemplation, contemplation, preparation, action, and maintenance. Before you get into the preparation stage, it's time to reframe how you think about your diabetes diagnosis. You now know that your future is in your control, so you can enter a space that allows self-care.

FOOD AND YOUR SOCIAL LIFE

As I've said before, eating well with diabetes simply means adopting a healthy way of eating—one that anyone can benefit from. Please don't feel as if you have to eat completely different food, which would require you to decline social invitations, skip dinner parties, or miss special family gatherings. This is (thankfully!) not the case.

Think about how you view social gatherings and the food available during those gatherings. You can refocus on quality time with loved ones, social connections, and the experience rather than the food, while knowing that no one food is forever off-limits.

If you tell yourself that you can't have your daughter's birthday cake, or your grandmother's popular mac and cheese, or whatever that special food might be, you are likely going to crave it more. Instead, consider a plan before you arrive at the social event so you can make a confident, informed decision that works with your personal diabetes management plan. That may mean checking your blood sugar and making a decision whether to have a healthy (smaller) portion, have a few bites, or abstain entirely. This will become easier as time goes on, and don't be surprised if you inspire other friends and family members to make healthier decisions as they see your lifestyle change.

FOOD AND EMOTIONS

Physical hunger is not the only reason people eat. Stress, boredom, anxiety, habit—there are so many reasons we may find ourselves eating when we're not actually hungry. Emotional eating—eating to satisfy our emotions rather than physical hunger—may also be an important factor to address. If you suspect you are an emotional eater, consider keeping a journal of how you feel when you eat. Notice if you are making different choices based on your emotions. Notice if certain people, situations, or feelings trigger you to make decisions about food that you wouldn't otherwise make.

Once you identify the triggers, you will be able to create a plan to either avoid those triggers or find a better solution when they occur. For example, do you ever find yourself bored after dinner and looking for more food, even though you aren't hungry? Think of three things unrelated to food that you can try instead. I've had clients make a cup of warm tea, take a relaxing bath, or go for a walk. It doesn't matter what it is, as long as it is enjoyable to you.

FOOD AND RELATIONSHIPS

As you start to make changes to the way you eat, think about whether you have any relationships that have food as their foundation. Is food the way your spouse, friends, or family members show their love? Do you see certain friends only at happy hour or brunch? This is not a problem, and as I've said before, it doesn't mean you need to decline any social invitations. It's simply something to be aware of. Maybe you want to let these people know about the changes you are making so that they will know how to best support you on your journey.

Consider Meditation

For years, when I heard the word *meditation* I thought about Buddhist monks or yogis, living apart and sitting still for hours. It seemed anything but relaxing. But meditation is actually one of the oldest ways to relax and reduce stress levels.

Meditation is a useful tool for calming the mind as well as the body. It is accessible to anyone, anywhere, making this a great addition to any health plan. Since we know that stress and anxiety can increase blood sugar levels, you may find it helpful to include a daily meditation practice in your own life.

To get started right away with meditation, try these simple steps:

1. Find a comfortable place in your home to sit or lie down.

2. Close your eyes and begin breathing naturally.

3. Focus your attention on how you feel—your body and your breath. Don't try to control your breath, simply focus on it. If your mind wanders, just gently refocus it on your breath.

4. Try this for only one or two minutes to begin with. Don't judge yourself; just refocus and keep going.

5. Start to incorporate this practice into your daily routine. Increase the length of time you meditate as you become more comfortable with it.

And if you are looking for more formal instruction, find out if local yoga studios offer a class, find a YouTube video online, or try the app HeadSpace.

Growing up in the South, I learned at an early age that food is often a way to show how much you care about someone, and I've made sure to always keep this perspective in my own personal relationships as well as my business. My hope is that you will also keep the love and enjoyment in your meals, and the people with whom you share them, while acknowledging how food plays a role in your relationships and having supportive conversations, if needed, where you explain to your loved ones exactly what you need and how they can help.

Rebuild Your Kitchen

Rebuilding your kitchen does not mean you need to go out and buy a lot of fancy, expensive equipment. It simply means setting you up for success by stocking it with the things that will enable you to make easy meals every day. That means the pantry items you'll use most often and the necessary tools to organize, prep, and cook your food. Having what you need on hand will make meal planning less time-consuming and will ensure that you're easily able to follow your diabetes nutrition guidelines every day—which will create the long-term results you are looking for.

THE PANTRY

The key to a well-stocked pantry is organization. While it may sound like simple advice, clearing out the clutter and stocking up on staples will ensure you always know what foods you have available and that you always have the basics on hand to whip up a quick meal any day of the week.

I recommend having several shelves, clear containers, bags, and baskets in your pantry so that you can easily see your groceries—no digging and shuffling required. Try to commit one or two minutes a day to maintaining your pantry's organization, as well. This will provide the additional bonus of helping you cut back on food waste.

Here is a list of staples that will be helpful to have on hand to get your pantry stocked for the recipes ahead.

- Almond butter
- Almonds, unsalted
- Anchovy paste
- Baking powder
- Barley, pearl
- Basil, dried
- Bay leaves
- Bread crumbs, gluten free
- Cashews
- Chia seeds
- Chili powder, chipotle
- Cherries, dried
- Cinnamon, ground
- Cloves, ground
- Cocoa powder, unsweetened
- Coconut flakes, unsweetened
- Coriander, ground
- Cornstarch
- Cumin, ground
- Curry powder
- Fennel seeds, ground
- Flaxseed, ground
- Flour, whole-wheat
- Garlic powder

- Ginger, ground
- Hemp seeds
- Honey
- Italian seasoning blend, dried
- Lentils, brown
- Maple syrup, pure
- Nonstick cooking spray (olive, coconut, or canola oil)
- Oats, quick
- Oats, rolled
- Oil, canola
- Oil, coconut
- Oil, olive
- Oil, sesame
- Onion, dried, minced
- Onion powder
- Oregano, dried
- Paprika, ground
- Peanut butter, unsalted, natural
- Peanuts, unsalted
- Pepitas (shelled, toasted pumpkin seeds)
- Pepper, cayenne, ground
- Pepper, red, crushed or flakes
- Peppercorns, black
- Peppercorns, white
- Quinoa
- Raisins, unsweetened
- Rice, brown
- Sage, dried, ground
- Salt
- Soy sauce, low sodium, gluten free
- Tahini
- Thyme, dried
- Walnuts
- Worcestershire sauce
- Vanilla extract, pure
- Vinegar, apple cider
- Vinegar, balsamic

- Vinegar, red wine
- Vinegar, rice wine

THE REFRIGERATOR

Having a clean and strategically stocked refrigerator will help you more than you might realize. Keeping it clutter free and clear of items that will not support your success will promote better outcomes for you, with the additional bonus of cutting down on food waste. Start with these staples to ensure you always have the building blocks for an easy, diabetes-friendly meal on hand.

- Eggs
- Favorite veggies, washed and chopped
- Fresh proteins such as fish and poultry (stored in the bottom drawer to prevent potential cross-contamination)
- Homemade salad dressings (perfect for marinades or quick salads; see chapter 14)
- Hummus, guacamole, salsa, or another favorite dip (see chapter 14 for homemade versions)
- Low-carb milk alternatives (unsweetened almond, coconut, or cashew)
- Low-sodium tamari, soy sauce, or coconut aminos (adds flavor without adding carbs)
- Mustard, whole-grain and Dijon (great for dressings)
- Plain yogurt (Greek yogurt is high in protein, but any plain yogurt is an easy add-in)
- Plant-based proteins such as precooked lentils and tofu
- Prewashed leafy greens (you're more likely to eat them when they're accessible and convenient)

THE FREEZER

It's no secret to those who know me that the frozen-foods section of the grocery store is one of my favorite aisles. When produce is frozen, it locks in nutrients at the peak of freshness, so it is always a healthy, affordable option. Keeping your freezer stocked with frozen veggies and lean proteins is the cornerstone of any well-planned diet.

In my signature diabetes management program, For the Love of Diabetes, I also recommend having backup pre-prepared meals at all times. This is any frozen meal that you can simply warm up and enjoy right away. It may be leftovers from a previous day or from making double portions. Think about freezing leftover healthy muffins, hearty soups, casseroles, and even dessert bites so that you always have a quick solution on hand.

I've often heard the misconception that eating healthy is expensive, but I can assure you that affordable improvements can be made to any eating plan. Buying frozen produce and cooking in large quantities to freeze for later are two effective cost-saving strategies.

Here are my favorite freezer staples that I always recommend having available:

- Salmon, shrimp, cod, and/or any other favorite seafood
- Dark chocolate (I always have a dark chocolate bar in my freezer to grab a square for a quick treat)
- Edamame (an easy high-protein snack for any time of the day)

- Frozen meat and poultry such as boneless chicken breasts, grass-fed beef, and lean ground turkey
- Frozen mixed berries (perfect for smoothies)
- Frozen vegetables (my favorites are spinach, broccoli, and green beans)
- Homemade frozen meals, snacks, and one-bite desserts
- Riced cauliflower (a quick low-carb side dish)

Plates, Utensils, and Cooking Equipment

Let me remind you that you certainly do not need a high-tech, expensive kitchen with all the newest types of cooking gadgets to succeed in your diabetes meal plan. Only basic equipment and basic cooking skills are required. But if you haven't cooked much before, there are several items you'll need to get started, and some things to think about.

First, look at how big your dishes are. Over the years, plates, cups, and bowls have gotten larger, and unknowingly with them, so have portion sizes. The standard dinner plate should be 9 inches across. It's a good idea to measure your plates and see how big they are. Also check your beverage glasses (4 to 8 ounces is standard) and any other dishes and bowls. Consider replacing extra-large dishes with more-appropriate-size ones to help give you all the possible advantages in the kitchen.

To make things as easy as possible, here's my quick checklist for some of the most helpful cooking equipment.

ESSENTIALS

- Food processor: for chopping and blending
- Blender (e.g., Ninja)
- Toaster
- Baking sheets: 18 by 13 inches
- Glass baking dishes: 8 inches square and 15 by 10 inches
- Garlic press
- Grater
- Good-quality knives: I recommend having a 3-inch paring knife and an 8-inch chef's knife
- Cutting boards: at least two—a plastic one for raw meats and a wooden one for cooked foods and/or veggies
- Digital food thermometer: to check cooked meats for proper internal temperature
- Measuring cups and spoons
- Storage containers and Sharpies: to store leftovers and mark the date to prevent food spoilage and reduce waste

NICE TO HAVE

- Slow cooker
- Instant Pot (electric pressure cooker): This new type of multicooker has nine functions including pressure cooker, slow cooker, and steamer
- Immersion blender: You can immerse this small blender on a stick right into a pot to purée soups and sauces without having to pour them back and forth
- Kitchen shears
- Spiralizer: a convenient kitchen tool used to cut veggies into noodlelike strips
- Ice cube trays: to freeze leftover herbs with olive oil or make fresh fruit/herb ice cubes to charge up your water
- Mandoline: a tool to slice foods easily into various cuts, including very thin slices
- Salad spinner
- Muffin tins

The Type 2 Diabetes Guide to Cooking and Enjoying Food

Having diabetes does not mean that you have to give up all your favorite foods. You may need to make some changes to your recipes to make them diabetes-friendly, but this is easily doable once you know how. Here are some tips that will help you maximize flavors, navigate ingredients, and energize your cooking while still managing your diabetes.

LEARN TO SPIRALIZE. A spiralizer is a simple tool that creates long, thin, noodlelike shreds of vegetables. This helps make zucchini, carrots, and other veggies easier to add to meals in a fun new way. No need to spend much money on this gadget; it can be found in grocery stores or online for less than $10.

ENLIST THE HELP OF YOUR FAVORITE HERBS AND SPICES. I want your food to be full of flavor so you look forward to every single meal. Instead of relying on salt and pepper to season your dishes, use fresh herbs and spices to give you loads of flavor. Keep fresh herbs growing in your kitchen, or at least maintain a well-stocked spice cabinet. Go beyond cinnamon, cilantro, and lemon and discover a world of fragrant seasonings waiting for you. Not only will these natural flavor enhancers add more variety to your meals, but they are also amazing sources of additional vitamins, nutrients, and antioxidants.

CREATE QUICK MARINADES, DRESSINGS, AND SAUCES. Diabetes-friendly meals should taste delicious. Bland and boring foods don't ever have to be part of your menu. Marinades, dressings, and sauces can be made in less than five minutes and stored in the refrigerator for one to two weeks, making them one of the easiest ways to add flavor to your meals. Use your favorite combo of oil and vinegar, vinegar and herbs, oil and citrus—whatever you prefer. Store in airtight jars or containers so you can quickly add a burst of flavor to proteins, veggies before roasting, green salads, stir-fries, and more. Check out chapter 14 for more inspiration.

MAKE GOOD PROTEIN CHOICES. Lean proteins are the best choice and should be consumed with every meal to fuel your body. Tuna, chicken, turkey, and lean meat cuts, like flank steak and pork tenderloin, are some of the best animal proteins to add into your diet. Beans are a great source of protein, as well, but because they also contain carbohydrates, portion size is very important.

SUBSTITUTE STARCHES. Vegetables are a great substitute for grains and can easily replace many favorite starches in your diet. Think cauliflower rice, spaghetti squash, and zucchini noodles for some simple ideas that can transform your meals from out-of-bounds to perfect.

DON'T SKIMP ON SNACKS. Eating regularly is an important part of keeping your blood sugar balanced. Be sure to keep snacks on hand, especially for those unforeseen occurrences that can push back your day and make mealtimes later than planned. Having a handful of nuts and a small apple on hand is just what you need to make it to the next meal without a problem.

REACH FOR ALTERNATIVES. Nut flours, such as almond or hazelnut flour, are great for adding texture and flavor to a wide variety of savory and sweet dishes. Nut milks are perfect for adding creaminess to foods without the carbohydrates contained in dairy products. Be open to trying new things and seeing what works and doesn't work for you as you begin this new way of cooking.

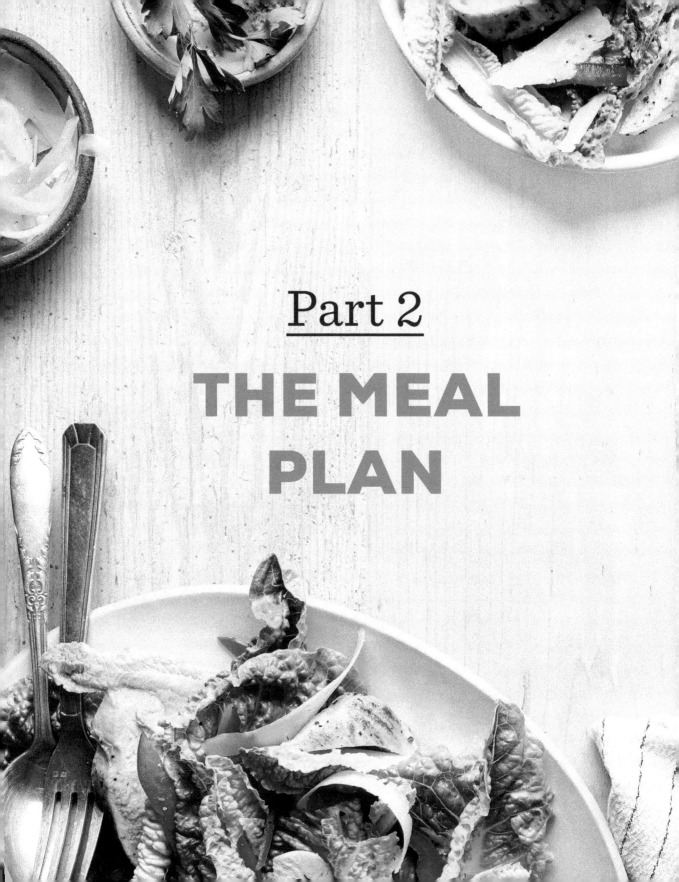

Part 2

THE MEAL PLAN

I CREATED THIS FOUR-WEEK PLAN as a straightforward guide to give you everything you need to lower your blood sugar levels right away, starting with the first meal! You will also be able to customize the meal plan to meet your personal preferences, since each recipe has a Complete the Plate feature to show you how to interchange recipes if you want. For example, if you don't like fish, you can simply swap out that recipe for a chicken or vegetarian recipe. Additionally, there are more than 100 recipes included in this cookbook, so you'll be sure to find the variety you are looking for.

Over the years, as I've created hundreds of meal plans for clients, I've noticed many of them ask for the same things. I've been sure to include those common requests in the meal plans you will see in chapter 4. Accessible ingredients, affordable foods, using up leftovers, all without having to spend *too* much time in the kitchen—please know I have incorporated all these things when creating the meal plans in this book. My intention is for these meal plans to be realistic for you, whether you are retired or are working long hours, because no one has the time to cook three meals every day.

I'll be sure to offer quick meal-prep tips to give you as many advantages and shortcuts in the kitchen as possible. However, it is important to acknowledge that preparing meals at home does require a time commitment, especially if you are used to dining out or grabbing food on the run most days of the week.

In chapter 5, I'll give you the best tips to stay on track year-round. From what to eat at your favorite restaurant to how to succeed while on vacation, you'll learn how to make this new way of eating work for you in any situation you may find yourself in.

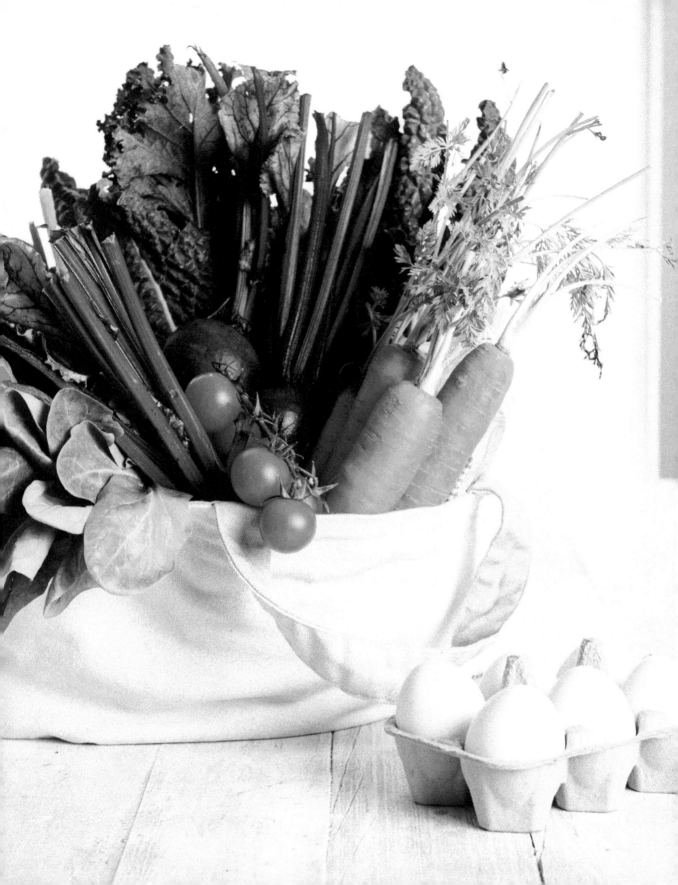

4

The Four-Week Plan for the Newly Diagnosed

This meal plan is full of delicious, nourishing foods that will begin to improve your health from the inside out. Plan and prepare as much as you can to help set yourself up for success and get yourself on the right track. And remember, this isn't about calorie counting; it's about creating the balance of nutrients your body needs—vegetables, healthy fats, energizing proteins, and high-fiber complex carbohydrates.

You'll notice that the plan includes a snack after every meal. As I point out in my diabetes management program, For the Love of Diabetes, snacks should be eaten about 2 to 3 hours after your main meals. If you are hungry less than 2 hours after a meal, you will likely need to evaluate whether you are eating balanced, satisfying meals. If it has been between 2 and 3 hours since your last meal, focus on snacks that are low in carbs: nonstarchy veggies, proteins, and healthy fats. If it has been more than 3 to 4 hours since your last meal, include at least 1 serving of carbs (15 grams of carbs) in addition to a veggie, protein, and/or healthy fat.

Having a snack after dinner can be helpful if eaten at least an hour or more before you go to sleep. Since it is recommended to avoid going more than 10 hours without eating, a bedtime snack containing 15 to 20 grams of carbs, combined with a protein, prevents the liver from releasing stored glucose in the bloodstream and assists in the management of fasting blood sugars the next morning.

Week 1

The first day and week of anything new can feel challenging. During this first week, I encourage you to draw inspiration from the results that will soon follow.

This week you will begin to retrain your taste buds to crave less sugar and less salt. As you begin to cook more balanced meals at home and increase the quality of the foods you are eating, you will resensitize your taste buds and foods will start to taste sweeter. Your taste buds regenerate approximately

every 10 to 12 days, so after this week you will be more than halfway there!

WEEK 1 SHOPPING LIST

Before you head to the grocery store, be sure to check that you also have the pantry staples listed in chapter 3. You'll need them for every week, and they do not appear in this shopping list.

CANNED AND BOTTLED ITEMS

- Almond milk, unsweetened, plain (1 pint)
- Applesauce, unsweetened (8 ounces)
- Artichoke hearts (1 [14-ounce] can)
- Black beans, low-sodium (2 [15-ounce] cans)
- Coconut milk, unsweetened, plain (1 pint)
- Chicken broth, low-sodium (1 quart)
- Enchilada sauce (1 [10-ounce] can)
- Sun-dried tomatoes (½ ounce)
- Thai red curry paste (1 [4-ounce] jar)
- Tomatoes, whole (1 [28-ounce] can)
- Vegetable broth, low-sodium (1 quart)

DAIRY AND EGGS

- Cheese, cheddar, shredded (3 ounces)
- Cheese, mozzarella, shredded (1 ounce)
- Cheese, string (5 pieces)
- Cottage cheese, low-fat (1 pint)
- Eggs (18)
- Goat cheese, crumbled (5 ounces)
- Greek yogurt, plain, nonfat (1 quart plus 6 ounces)
- Yogurt, unsweetened, vanilla, nonfat (6 ounces)

FROZEN FOODS

- Cauliflower (16 ounces)

MEAT AND FISH

- Canadian bacon (2 ounces)
- Chicken breasts, boneless, skinless (2)
- Chicken legs (6)
- Salmon fillet (1 pound)
- Shrimp (8 ounces)
- Trout, whole, cleaned, deboned (2)

FRESH PRODUCE

- Apples (2)
- Arugula (1 ounce)
- Avocados (3)
- Beet (1)
- Bell pepper, green (1)
- Bell peppers, red (4)
- Berries, mixed (2 pints)
- Blueberries (1 pint)
- Brussels sprouts (1 pound)
- Carrots (1 bunch)
- Cauliflower (1 head)
- Cilantro, fresh (1 bunch)
- Cucumber (1)
- Dill, fresh (1 bunch)
- Garlic (2 heads)
- Kale (1 bunch)
- Lemons (5)
- Lettuce, leaf (1 head)
- Limes (2)
- Microgreens (1 ounce)
- Mint, fresh (1 bunch)
- Mushrooms, brown (12 ounces)

- Mushrooms, shiitake (2 or 3)
- Onion, red (1)
- Onions, yellow (5)
- Parsley, fresh (1 bunch)
- Peaches (2)
- Pepper, jalapeño (1)
- Pepper, poblano (1)
- Rosemary, fresh (1 bunch)
- Scallions (1 bunch)
- Spinach (5 ounces)
- Squash, spaghetti (1)
- Thyme, fresh (1 bunch)
- Tomato, roma (1)
- Tomatoes, cherry (1 pint)
- Vegetables for roasting such as broccoli, asparagus, bell peppers, onions, cauliflower (4 cups)
- Vegetables for snacking such as cauliflower, radishes, cucumbers, bell peppers (5 cups)
- Zucchini, small (8)

OTHER ITEMS

- Bread, whole-wheat, thin-sliced (1 loaf)
- Chocolate, dark, at least 70 percent cocoa (1 small bar)
- Chocolate chips, dark, at least 70 percent cocoa (1 ½ ounces)
- Corn tortillas, 6-inch (4)
- Hummus (8 ounces)
- Pistachios, unsalted, in-shell (16-ounce bag)
- Pita bread, whole-grain (2)
- Wine, red, dry

PREP FOR WEEK 1

These are time-saving strategies to set you up for success for the week ahead. Prepare these foods on the weekend so you will have grab-and-go options throughout the week.

- Make Breakfast Egg Bites (page 80)
- Make Chocolate-Zucchini Muffins (page 76)
- Make Chicken Tortilla Soup (page 97)
- Make Oat and Walnut Granola (page 75) —one batch will be enough for the whole month

Calorie and Carb Add-Ins

These calorie and carb add-ins are a way for you to customize your meal plan to meet your specific needs and preferences. If you feel you need more food without the carbs, choose the add-ins with fewer than 5 grams of carbs. If more carbs are okay in your personal daily meals, feel free to choose the add-ins with 10 to 20 grams of carbs. You can use this list for all four weeks of your meal plan.

100 TO 150 CALORIES WITH 10 TO 20 GRAMS OF CARBS

- ½ cup cooked quinoa
- 6 ounces plain nonfat Greek yogurt
- ½ cup shelled edamame
- ¼ cup hummus
- ½ cup black beans
- 1 ounce dark chocolate (½ ounce equals 1 to 2 squares)
- 1 cup cooked winter squash
- ¾ cup cooked green peas
- ¾ cup cooked oatmeal
- 1½ cups raspberries

100 TO 150 CALORIES WITH FEWER THAN 5 GRAMS OF CARBS

- 1 tablespoon natural nut butter
- 2 tablespoons unsalted nuts
- 2 hard-boiled eggs
- 2 cups nonstarchy vegetables
- 1 to 2 ounces natural cheese
- 1 tablespoon olive or coconut oil
- ½ avocado
- ½ cup tofu
- ½ cup cottage cheese
- 3 ounces grilled chicken

MONDAY

Breakfast	Chocolate-Zucchini Muffin (page 76) Greek Yogurt Sundae (page 73)
Snack	¼ cup walnuts, 1 piece string cheese, and ½ apple
Lunch	Chicken Tortilla Soup (page 97) Cucumber, Tomato, and Avocado Salad (page 101)
Snack	½ apple with 1 tablespoon almond butter
Dinner	Black Bean Enchilada Skillet Casserole (page 135) topped with ¼ sliced avocado Spicy Roasted Cauliflower with Lime (page 124)
Snack	Leftover Chocolate-Zucchini Muffins and 2 tablespoons walnuts

TUESDAY

Breakfast	2 Breakfast Egg Bites (page 80) Leftover Chocolate-Zucchini Muffins, ½ cup plain nonfat Greek yogurt
Snack	½ cup blueberries and 1 piece string cheese
Lunch	Leftover Cucumber, Tomato, and Avocado Salad Leftover Black Bean Enchilada Skillet Casserole
Snack	¼ cup walnuts and 1 cup favorite nonstarchy veggies with 2 tablespoons hummus
Dinner	Easy Chicken Cacciatore (page 160) Mozzarella and Artichoke Stuffed Spaghetti Squash (page 142)
Snack	1 ounce pistachios (49 nuts)

WEDNESDAY

Breakfast	1 serving Oat and Walnut Granola (page 75) 1 cup plain nonfat Greek yogurt
Snack	Leftover Chocolate-Zucchini Muffins and 1 piece string cheese
Lunch	Leftover Chicken Tortilla Soup topped with ¼ sliced avocado ⅓ cup black beans, Leftover Spicy Roasted Cauliflower with Lime
Snack	2 cups favorite nonstarchy vegetables with ¼ cup hummus
Dinner	Roasted Salmon with Honey-Mustard Sauce (page 194) 2 cups favorite roasted vegetables (cook alongside the salmon) ½ cup cooked quinoa
Snack	½ ounce dark chocolate and 2 tablespoons favorite nuts

THURSDAY

Breakfast	2 leftover Breakfast Egg Bites Leftover Chocolate-Zucchini Muffins ½ cup plain nonfat Greek yogurt
Snack	¼ cup walnuts and ½ cup favorite berries
Lunch	Leftover Black Bean Enchilada Skillet Casserole topped with ¼ sliced avocado Leftover Spicy Roasted Cauliflower with Lime
Snack	1 small apple with 1 tablespoon almond butter
Dinner	Leftover Easy Chicken Cacciatore Leftover Mozzarella and Artichoke Stuffed Spaghetti Squash Bowls
Snack	1 ounce pistachios (49 nuts)

FRIDAY

Breakfast	½ Coconut-Berry Sunrise Smoothie (page 72) 2 leftover Breakfast Egg Bites
Snack	½ cup blueberries and 1 piece string cheese
Lunch	Leftover Chicken Tortilla Soup topped with ¼ sliced avocado ⅓ cup black beans Simple green salad with Ranch Vegetable Dip and Dressing (page 239) or other healthy dressing
Snack	Leftover Chocolate-Zucchini Muffins and ¼ cup walnuts
Dinner	Leftover Roasted Salmon with Honey-Mustard Sauce 2 cups favorite roasted vegetables, ½ cup cooked quinoa
Dessert (optional)	Grilled Peach and Coconut Yogurt Bowls (page 221)

SATURDAY

Breakfast	Brussels Sprout Hash and Eggs (page 84) 1 cup favorite berries
Snack	Leftover Chocolate-Zucchini Muffins and 1 piece string cheese
Lunch	Thai Peanut, Carrot, and Shrimp Soup (page 95) Red Pepper, Goat Cheese, and Arugula Open-Faced Grilled Sandwich (page 113)
Snack	Leftover Coconut-Berry Sunrise Smoothie
Dinner	Beet, Goat Cheese, and Walnut Pesto with Zoodles (page 132)
Dessert (optional):	Leftover Grilled Peach and Coconut Yogurt Bowl

SUNDAY

Breakfast	Crispy Breakfast Pita with Egg and Canadian Bacon (page 82) topped with ¼ sliced avocado ½ cup favorite berries
Snack	Leftover Brussels Sprout Hash and Eggs
Lunch	Leftover Thai Peanut, Carrot, and Shrimp Soup Red Pepper, Goat Cheese, and Arugula Open-Faced Grilled Sandwich (page 113)
Snack	½ pita bread and 2 cups favorite nonstarchy vegetables with 2 tablespoons Ranch Vegetable Dip and Dressing
Dinner	Whole Veggie-Stuffed Trout (page 201)
Snack	½ cup plain nonfat Greek yogurt with 2 tablespoons crushed walnuts, 1 teaspoon ground cinnamon, and 2 tablespoons favorite berries

Week 2

Congratulations on reaching week 2! As you start the second week, you should notice an improvement in blood sugar levels already, if you are monitoring at home. Many of my clients will mention that they're surprised at how satisfying the meals are when they are paired properly, and I hope you are finding this to be true as well. Eating the *right* combination of *real* foods will produce success over and over again.

Remember, this isn't a diet. You are simply making sure you are giving your body the balance of macronutrients that it needs to function optimally, while being strategic in the type and amount of carbohydrates you eat to help lower your blood sugar levels.

This is a good week to check in with yourself to make sure you are drinking enough water throughout the day. The daily meal plans provided have the recommended amount of fiber, but many people eat far less fiber before they start to improve the way they eat. Maintaining adequate hydration levels will give your body the ability to fully digest your food and increase mental clarity and energy levels as you continue forward.

WEEK 2 SHOPPING LIST

CANNED AND BOTTLED ITEMS

- Almond milk, unsweetened, plain (1 pint)
- Artichoke hearts (1 [14-ounce] can)
- Beef broth, low-sodium (1 quart)
- Coconut milk, unsweetened, plain (1 pint)
- Pesto (2 ounces)
- Tomatoes, crushed (1 [28-ounce] can)
- Tomatoes, whole (1 [28-ounce] can)
- Tomato paste (3 [6-ounce] cans)
- Tuna, chunk light, packed in water (1 [5-ounce] can)
- Vegetable broth, low-sodium (1 quart)

DAIRY AND EGGS

- Cheese, cheddar, shredded (2 ounces)
- Cheese, mozzarella, shredded (1 ounce)
- Cheese, natural, any type (3 ounces)
- Cheese, string (3 pieces)
- Eggs (12)
- Goat cheese, crumbled (3 ounces)
- Greek yogurt, plain, nonfat (1 pint)
- Yogurt, unsweetened, vanilla, nonfat (6 ounces)

FROZEN FOODS

- Berries, mixed (16 ounces)
- Cauliflower (16 ounces)
- Spinach (1 [10-ounce] package)

MEAT AND FISH

- Beef stew meat (1 pound)
- Chicken breast, cooked (12 ounces)
- Salmon fillet (1 pound)
- Tilapia (8 ounces)
- Turkey, lean, ground (1 pound)

FRESH PRODUCE

- Apples (2)
- Asparagus (1 pound)
- Arugula (1 ounce)
- Avocados (3)
- Bean sprouts (4 ounces)
- Bell peppers, red (4)
- Berries, mixed (2 pints)

- Blueberries (1 pint)
- Broccoli (4 heads)
- Cabbage, green (1 small head)
- Carrots (1 bunch)
- Celery (1 bunch)
- Cilantro, fresh (1 bunch)
- Dill, fresh (1 bunch)
- Fruit of choice (2)
- Garlic (3 heads)
- Ginger (1 small knob)
- Kale, baby (10 ounces)
- Leafy greens such as kale and/or spinach (2 ounces)
- Lemons (2)
- Lettuce, leaf (2 heads)
- Limes (2)
- Mango (1)
- Mushrooms, brown (1¼ pounds)
- Onion, red (1)
- Onion, white (1)
- Onions, yellow (6)
- Parsley, fresh (1 bunch)
- Pepper, jalapeño (1)
- Scallions (1 bunch)
- Spinach (3 bunches)
- Squash, delicata (1)

- Sweet potatoes (4)
- Tomatoes (1 small, 1 large)
- Tomatoes, cherry (1 pint)
- Vegetables for snacking such as cauliflower, radishes, cucumbers, bell peppers (10 cups)

OTHER ITEMS

- Bread, whole-wheat, thin-sliced (1 loaf)
- Chocolate, dark, at least 70 percent cocoa (1 small bar)
- Flatbread, whole-wheat (2)
- Hummus (8 ounces)
- Tortilla, 8-inch, whole-wheat, low carb (4)

PREP FOR WEEK 2

- Make Spinach, Artichoke, and Goat Cheese Breakfast Bake (page 85)
- Make tuna salad for Tomato Tuna Melts (page 192)
- Bake sweet potatoes
- Make Tomato and Kale Soup (page 91)
- Make Ranch Vegetable Dip and Dressing (page 239)
- Make Easy Italian Dressing (page 238)

Breakfast	2 servings Spinach, Artichoke, and Goat Cheese Breakfast Bake (page 85) 1 small baked sweet potato topped with 2 tablespoons crushed nuts (almonds, pecans, walnuts)
Snack	2 cups favorite nonstarchy vegetables with ¼ cup Quick Guacamole (page 233)
Lunch	Tomato Tuna Melts (page 192) Tomato and Kale Soup (page 91)
Snack	½ cup berries and ¼ cup walnuts
Dinner	Lentil Loaf (page 148) Simple green salad with Ranch Vegetable Dip and Dressing (page 239)
Snack	1 ounce natural cheese and 1 cup sliced veggies with 2 tablespoons hummus

TUESDAY

Breakfast	1 serving Oat and Walnut Granola (page 75) 1 cup plain nonfat Greek yogurt
Snack	1 cup berries and 1 piece string cheese
Lunch	Leftover Lentil Loaf Simple green salad with Ranch Vegetable Dip and Dressing
Snack	½ apple with 2 tablespoons almond butter
Dinner	Beef and Mushroom Barley Soup (page 99) Roasted Asparagus, Onions, and Red Peppers (page 126)
Snack	1 ounce natural cheese and 1 cup sliced vegetables with 2 tablespoons hummus

WEEK 2

WEDNESDAY

Breakfast	2 servings Spinach, Artichoke, and Goat Cheese Breakfast Bake ½ Coconut-Berry Sunrise Smoothie (page 72)
Snack	2 cups favorite nonstarchy vegetables with ¼ cup Quick Guacamole (page 233)
Lunch	Leftover Tomato Tuna Melt Leftover Tomato and Kale Soup
Snack	1 apple with 2 tablespoons almond butter
Dinner	Leftover Lentil Loaf Leftover Roasted Asparagus, Onions, and Red Peppers
Snack	½ ounce dark chocolate and 2 tablespoons almonds or other favorite nuts

THURSDAY

Breakfast	2 servings leftover Spinach, Artichoke, and Goat Cheese Breakfast Bake 1 small baked sweet potato topped with cinnamon and 2 table-spoons crushed nuts (pecans, walnuts, almonds)
Snack	Leftover Coconut-Berry Sunrise Smoothie
Lunch	Leftover Beef and Mushroom Barley Soup Simple green salad with Easy Italian Dressing (page 238)
Snack	¼ cup walnuts and 1 piece string cheese ½ cup Roasted Delicata Squash (page 125)
Dinner	Ginger-Glazed Salmon and Broccoli (page 195) Leftover Roasted Delicata Squash
Snack	½ ounce dark chocolate and ¼ cup nuts

Breakfast
Avocado and Goat Cheese Toast (page 74)
topped with 1 poached egg
½ cup berries

Snack
Leftover Tomato and Kale Soup

Lunch
Leftover Lentil Loaf
Simple green salad with Easy Italian Dressing

Snack
1 piece string cheese and 1 small fruit of choice

Dinner
Leftover Beef and Mushroom Barley Soup
Red Pepper, Goat Cheese, and Arugula Open-Faced Grilled Sandwich
(page 113)

Snack
1 ounce pistachios (49 nuts)

SATURDAY

Breakfast
2 servings Sweet Potato, Onion, and Turkey Sausage Hash (page 87)
Hard-boiled or poached egg

Snack
Leftover Tomato and Kale Soup

Lunch
Thai-Style Chicken Roll-Ups (page 116)
Simple green salad with Easy Italian Dressing

Snack
1 ounce natural cheese and 1 cup sliced vegetables with
2 tablespoons hummus

Dinner
Mushroom and Pesto Flatbread Pizza (page 134)
Sautéed Spinach and Tomatoes (page 120)

Dessert (optional)
Berry Smoothie Pops (page 220)

SUNDAY	
Breakfast	Leftover Sweet Potato, Onion, and Turkey Sausage Hash
Snack	2 cups vegetables with ¼ cup Quick Guacamole
Lunch	Leftover Thai-Style Chicken Roll-Up 1 small fruit of choice Simple green salad with Easy Italian Dressing
Snack	½ cup plain nonfat Greek yogurt with 2 tablespoons crushed walnuts, 1 teaspoon cinnamon, and 2 tablespoons berries
Dinner	Blackened Tilapia with Mango Salsa (page 206) Roasted Lemon and Garlic Broccoli (page 122) ½ cup quinoa
Snack	½ cup blueberries and 2 tablespoons favorite nuts

Week 3

As you enter week 3, I hope you are starting to feel your confidence grow! Be proud of your success thus far and how you've taken the steps to implement a new way of eating for the betterment of your long-term health. If you haven't followed the meal plans exactly, it's okay. You don't have to eat perfectly to get results; you simply have to improve on where you started and continue to push forward. Consistency and balance are the keys to success.

By now you should be able to identify new favorite meals, snacks, and foods that you enjoy and you know are "safe" in the sense that they will not raise your blood sugar. Having these go-to options will serve you again and again, because you know you can always come back to them throughout your diabetes journey.

Be sure to check in with yourself to acknowledge the changes you are experiencing—both physical and emotional. If you find it helpful, jot down notes and observations in the meal plan, since it is yours to customize.

WEEK 3 SHOPPING LIST

CANNED AND BOTTLED ITEMS

- Almond milk, unsweetened, plain (1 pint)
- Black beans, low-sodium (1 [15-ounce] can)
- Coconut milk, canned (1 [15-ounce] can)
- Chickpeas, low-sodium (1 [15-ounce] can)
- Coconut milk, unsweetened, plain (1 pint)
- Sun-dried tomatoes (½ ounce)
- Tomato paste (2 [6-ounce] cans)
- Tomatoes, whole (1 [28-ounce] can)

- Tuna, chunk light, packed in water (1 [5-ounce] can)
- Vegetable broth, low-sodium (1 quart)
- White beans, low-sodium (1 [15-ounce] can)

DAIRY AND EGGS

- Butter (1 stick)
- Cheese, natural, any variety (1 ounce)
- Cheese, Parmesan, grated (5 ounces)
- Cheese, string (3 pieces)
- Cottage cheese, low-fat (8 ounces)
- Eggs (18)
- Goat cheese, crumbled (2 ounces)
- Greek yogurt, plain, nonfat (1 quart)
- Yogurt, unsweetened, vanilla, nonfat (6 ounces)

MEAT AND FISH

- Canadian bacon (1 ounce)
- Chicken breast, boneless, skinless (1 [8-ounce] breast)
- Protein, lean, any type (8 ounces)
- Salmon (4 [4-ounce] fillets)
- Sea scallops (1 pound)
- Shrimp, peeled, deveined (1 pound)
- Turkey, lean, ground (8 ounces)
- Turkey, sliced (1 ounce) (optional)

FRESH PRODUCE

- Apples (2)
- Asparagus (1 pound)
- Avocados (3)
- Basil, fresh (1 bunch)
- Bell peppers, red (4)
- Berries, mixed (2 pints)
- Blueberries (1 pint)

- Brussels sprouts (1 pound)
- Cabbage, green (1 small head)
- Cabbage, red (1 small head)
- Carrots (2 bunches)
- Celery (1 bunch)
- Cilantro, fresh (1 bunch)
- Cucumbers (2)
- Garlic (2 heads)
- Ginger (1 small knob)
- Jicama (1 small)
- Leafy greens such as kale and/or spinach (2 ounces)
- Lemons (4)
- Lettuce, leaf (2 heads)
- Lettuce, romaine hearts (2 heads)
- Limes (3)
- Mango (1)
- Mint, fresh (1 bunch)
- Mushrooms, brown (2 ounces)
- Onion, red (1)
- Onions, yellow (2)
- Pear (1)
- Peppers, jalapeño (2)
- Salad greens, mixed (10 ounces)
- Scallions (2 bunches)

- Spinach (1 bunch)
- Spinach, baby (1 ounce)
- Sweet potato (1)
- Tomatillos (8 ounces)
- Tomato (1)
- Tomatoes, cherry (1 pint)
- Vegetables for snacking such as cauliflower, radishes, cucumbers, bell peppers (7 cups)

OTHER ITEMS

- Bread, whole-wheat, thin-sliced (1 loaf)
- Chocolate, dark, at least 70 percent cocoa (1 small bar)
- Dinner rolls, whole-wheat (4)
- Pita bread, whole-wheat (4)
- Wine, white, dry

PREP FOR WEEK 3

- Make Breakfast Egg Bites (page 80)
- Make hummus for Tuna, Hummus, and Veggie Wraps (page 115)
- Make Curried Carrot Soup (page 94)
- Make Easy Italian Dressing (page 238)

MONDAY

Breakfast	2 Breakfast Egg Bites (page 80) in whole-wheat pita with a handful of favorite greens ½ Coconut-Berry Sunrise Smoothie (page 72)
Snack	½ apple with 1 tablespoon almond butter
Lunch	Tuna, Hummus, and Veggie Wraps (page 115) with 2 slices avocado Curried Carrot Soup (page 94)
Snack	½ apple and 1 piece string cheese
Dinner	Barbecue Turkey Burger Sliders (page 170) Cabbage Slaw Salad (page 102) Simple green salad with Easy Italian Dressing (page 238)
Snack	¼ cup leftover hummus with 2 cups favorite veggies

TUESDAY

Breakfast	Greek Yogurt Sundae (page 73) 1 serving Oat and Walnut Granola (page 75)
Snack	¼ cup walnuts
Lunch	Leftover Tuna, Hummus, and Veggie Wraps with 2 slices avocado Leftover Curried Carrot Soup
Snack	Leftover Coconut-Berry Sunrise Smoothie
Dinner	Roasted Salmon with Salsa Verde (page 197) Rainbow Black Bean Salad (page 106)
Snack	½ ounce dark chocolate crumbled over ½ cup plain nonfat Greek yogurt and 1 tablespoon crushed nuts sprinkled with cinnamon

WEDNESDAY

Breakfast	2 leftover Breakfast Egg Bites ½ cup blueberries and ½ cup plain nonfat Greek yogurt 1 serving Oat and Walnut Granola
Snack	2 tablespoons leftover hummus with 1 cup cut vegetables
Lunch	Leftover Barbecue Turkey Burger Sliders, 1 baked sweet potato with 1 teaspoon olive oil, Simple green salad with Easy Italian Dressing
Snack	1 piece string cheese and 1 small pear
Dinner	Shrimp Burgers with Fruity Salsa and Salad (page 215) Leftover Rainbow Black Bean Salad
Snack	½ pita stuffed with Dijon mustard, 1 ounce natural cheese, 1 cup favorite veggies, and 1 ounce sliced turkey (optional)

THURSDAY

Breakfast	Avocado and Goat Cheese Toast (page 74) 2 leftover Breakfast Egg Bites
Snack	2 tablespoons leftover hummus with 1 cup cut vegetables
Lunch	Leftover Roasted Salmon with Salsa Verde Leftover Rainbow Black Bean Salad Simple green salad with Easy Italian Dressing
Snack	½ cup berries, ½ cup plain nonfat Greek yogurt, and 2 tablespoons nuts
Dinner	Chicken Caesar Salad (page 154) Leftover Curried Carrot Soup 1 whole-wheat pita, broiled for 1 to 2 minutes
Snack	¼ cup almonds or favorite nuts Dessert (optional): 1 or 2 Chocolate Peanut Butter Freezer Bites (page 222)

FRIDAY

Breakfast	1 serving Oat and Walnut Granola with 1 cup plain nonfat Greek yogurt
Snack	½ apple with 1 tablespoon almond butter
Lunch	Leftover Chicken Caesar Salad 2 tablespoons hummus with 1 whole-wheat pita
Snack	¼ cup nuts of choice
Dinner	Leftover Shrimp Burgers with Fruity Salsa and Salad Leftover Rainbow Black Bean Salad
Snack	½ cup cooked oatmeal + 1 ½ teaspoons chia seeds + 1 tablespoon favorite crushed nuts

SATURDAY

Breakfast	Gluten-Free Carrot and Oat Pancakes (page 78) 1 scrambled egg
Snack	½ cup berries and ¼ cup favorite nuts
Lunch	Leftover Chicken Caesar Salad Crispy Parmesan Cups with White Beans and Veggies (page 136)
Snack	½ apple with 1 tablespoon almond butter
Dinner	4 ounces favorite grilled protein, ½ cup starch (quinoa, beans), and 2 cups vegetables with 2 tablespoons Easy Italian Dressing
Dessert (optional)	1 or 2 leftover Chocolate Peanut Butter Freezer Bites

Breakfast	Brussels Sprout Hash and Eggs (page 84) 1 cup berries 1 slice Canadian bacon
Snack	½ recipe Coconut-Berry Sunrise Smoothie (page 72)
Lunch:	Leftover Crispy Parmesan Cups with White Beans and Veggies 4 ounces favorite lean protein Simple green salad with Easy Italian Dressing topped with 3 slices avocado
Snack	¼ cup walnuts, 1 piece string cheese, and ½ cup berries
Dinner	Scallops and Asparagus Skillet (page 208) ½ cup cooked quinoa
Snack	½ ounce dark chocolate crumbled over ½ cup plain nonfat Greek yogurt and 1 tablespoon crushed nuts sprinkled with cinnamon

WEEK 3

Week 4

So much can change in just a few weeks, and I hope you are continuing to feel encouraged as you understand that a diabetes diagnosis does not mean bland, boring food. Well done on your success so far!

As you finish the final week of this four-week meal plan, know that this is just the beginning. As you become more aware of which dishes you prefer and what works best for your blood sugar levels, things will continue to get easier and easier. Because you have followed this meal plan, you have been teaching yourself more about what your body needs and have likely noticed what it has been missing as well.

With all of this in mind, be sure to stay tuned in to your expectations and make sure they remain realistic. Always acknowledge how far you've come, while being consistent in your goal to manage your diabetes.

WEEK 4 SHOPPING LIST

CANNED AND BOTTLED ITEMS

- Almond milk, unsweetened, plain (1 quart)
- Applesauce, unsweetened (4 ounces)
- Artichoke hearts (1 [14-ounce] can)
- Baby corn (1 [14-ounce] can)
- Chicken or vegetable broth, low-sodium (1 pint)
- Chickpeas, low-sodium (3 [15-ounce] cans)
- Coconut milk, unsweetened, plain (1 pint)
- Tomatoes, fire-roasted (1 [15-ounce] can)
- Tomatoes, whole (1 [28-ounce] can)

DAIRY AND EGGS

- Cheese, cheddar, shredded (2 ounces)
- Cheese, goat, crumbled (3 ounces)
- Cheese, mozzarella, shredded (1 ounce)
- Cheese, mozzarella, sliced (4 ounces)
- Cheese, natural, any type (3 ounces)
- Cheese, Parmesan, grated (1 ounce)
- Cheese, string (1 piece)
- Eggs (18)
- Greek yogurt, plain, nonfat (1 quart)
- Yogurt, unsweetened, vanilla, nonfat (6 ounces)

FROZEN FOODS

- Spinach (1 [10-ounce] package)

MEAT AND FISH

- Canadian bacon (2 ounces)
- Chicken breast, boneless, skinless (1 pound)
- Chicken legs (6)
- Salmon (4 [4-ounce] fillets)
- Turkey, lean, ground (1 pound)

FRESH PRODUCE

- Apple (1)
- Asparagus (2 pounds)
- Avocados (4)
- Basil, fresh (1 bunch)
- Bell peppers, red (3)
- Berries, mixed (2 pints)
- Blueberries (1 pint)
- Bok choy (1 head)
- Broccoli (2 heads)
- Carrots (2)
- Cilantro, fresh (1 bunch)
- Cucumber (1)

- Fruit of choice (1)
- Garlic (2 heads)
- Ginger (1 small knob)
- Kale, baby (4 ounces)
- Leafy greens such as kale and/or spinach (2 ounces)
- Lemons (2)
- Lettuce, leaf (2 heads)
- Limes (2)
- Microgreens (1 ounce)
- Mint, fresh (1 bunch)
- Mushrooms, brown (8 ounces)
- Mushrooms, shiitake (4 ounces)
- Onion, red (1)
- Onion, white (1)
- Onion, yellow (1)
- Oregano, fresh (1 bunch)
- Parsley, fresh (1 bunch)
- Pear (1)
- Scallions (1 bunch)
- Spinach (6 ounces)
- Squash, butternut (1)
- Squash, delicata (1)
- Sweet potato (1)
- Tomatoes (3 large, 1 small)

- Vegetables for roasting such as broccoli, asparagus, bell peppers, onions, cauliflower (1 cup)
- Vegetables for snacking such as cauliflower, radishes, cucumbers, bell peppers (5 cups)
- Zucchini (2 small)

OTHER ITEMS

- Bread, whole-wheat, thin-sliced (1 loaf)
- Chocolate, dark, at least 70 percent cocoa (1 small bar)
- Chocolate chips, dark, at least 70 percent cocoa (10 ounces)
- Hummus (8 ounces)
- Pita bread, whole-wheat (2)
- Tofu, firm (1 [14-ounce] container)

PREP FOR WEEK 4

- Make Chocolate-Zucchini Muffins (page 76)
- Make Falafel with Creamy Garlic-Yogurt Sauce (page 146)
- Make Quick Guacamole (page 233)

MONDAY

Breakfast	Chocolate-Zucchini Muffins (page 76) Coconut-Berry Sunrise Smoothie (page 72) 1 or 2 hard-boiled eggs
Snack	¼ cup walnuts and 1 fruit of choice
Lunch	Salmon, Quinoa, and Avocado Salad (page 111)
Snack	½ cup berries and ½ cup plain nonfat Greek yogurt with 2 teaspoons chia seeds and 1 teaspoon cinnamon
Dinner	Baked Tofu and Mixed Vegetable Bowl (page 140) ½ cup chickpeas
Snack	1 ounce natural cheese and ½ whole-wheat pita

TUESDAY

Breakfast	Greek Yogurt Sundae (page 73) 1 serving Oat and Walnut Granola (page 75)
Snack	½ cup mashed chickpeas and 1 cup vegetables seasoned with spice of choice
Lunch	Leftover Salmon, Quinoa, and Avocado Salad
Snack	Leftover Coconut-Berry Sunrise Smoothie
Dinner	Quick Weeknight Chicken Parmesan (page 158) Roasted Asparagus, Onions, and Red Peppers (page 126)
Snack	¼ cup favorite nuts and 1 tablespoon raisins or other unsweetened dried fruit

WEDNESDAY

Breakfast	Greek Yogurt Sundae (page 73) Leftover Chocolate-Zucchini Muffins
Snack	½ serving leftover Baked Tofu and Mixed Vegetable Bowl
Lunch	Falafel with Creamy Garlic-Yogurt Sauce (page 146), ¼ avocado, and 1 cup roasted vegetables
Snack	½ apple with 1 tablespoon almond butter
Dinner	Leftover Quick Weeknight Chicken Parmesan Leftover Roasted Asparagus, Onions, and Red Peppers
Snack	1 ounce natural cheese and 1 cup sliced vegetables with 2 tablespoons hummus

THURSDAY

Breakfast	Leftover Chocolate-Zucchini Muffins Coconut-Berry Sunrise Smoothie (page 72) 1 or 2 hard-boiled eggs
Snack	½ serving leftover Baked Tofu and Mixed Vegetable Bowl
Lunch	Sweet Potato, Chickpea, and Kale Bowl with Creamy Tahini Sauce (page 138)
Snack	Leftover Falafel with Creamy Garlic-Yogurt Sauce
Dinner	2 servings Turkey and Quinoa Caprese Casserole (page 172)
Snack	½ ounce dark chocolate and 2 tablespoons favorite nuts

WEEK 4

FRIDAY	
Breakfast	Avocado and Goat Cheese Toast (page 74) Leftover Chocolate-Zucchini Muffins
Snack	Leftover Coconut-Berry Sunrise Smoothie
Lunch	2 servings leftover Turkey and Quinoa Caprese Casserole
Snack	¼ cup Quick Guacamole (page 233) with 2 cups vegetables
Dinner	Leftover Sweet Potato, Chickpea, and Kale Bowl with Creamy Tahini Sauce
Dessert (optional)	1 or 2 Dark Chocolate Almond Butter Cups (page 223)

SATURDAY	
Breakfast	2 servings Spinach, Artichoke, and Goat Cheese Breakfast Bake (page 85) ½ cup blueberries with ½ cup plain nonfat Greek yogurt
Snack	¼ cup walnuts and leftover Chocolate-Zucchini Muffins
Lunch	Warm Barley and Squash Salad with Balsamic Vinaigrette (page 107) Spice-Rubbed Crispy Roast Chicken (page 155)
Snack	½ apple with 1 tablespoon almond butter
Dinner	Mushroom Cutlets with Creamy Sauce (page 144) Roasted Delicata Squash (page 125)
Snack	1 ounce natural cheese and 1 cup sliced vegetables with 2 tablespoons hummus
Dessert (optional)	1 or 2 Dark Chocolate Almond Butter Cups (page 223)

SUNDAY

Breakfast
Crispy Breakfast Pita with Egg and Canadian Bacon (page 82)
with 2 or 3 slices avocado
Leftover Chocolate-Zucchini Muffins

Snack
1 small pear and 1 piece string cheese

Lunch
Leftover Mushroom Cutlets with Creamy Sauce
Leftover Roasted Delicata Squash

Snack
½ cup berries

Dinner
Leftover Warm Barley and Squash Salad with Balsamic Vinaigrette
Leftover Spice-Rubbed Crispy Roast Chicken

Snack
½ cup plain nonfat Greek yogurt with 2 tablespoons crushed walnuts,
1 teaspoon cinnamon, and 2 tablespoons favorite berries

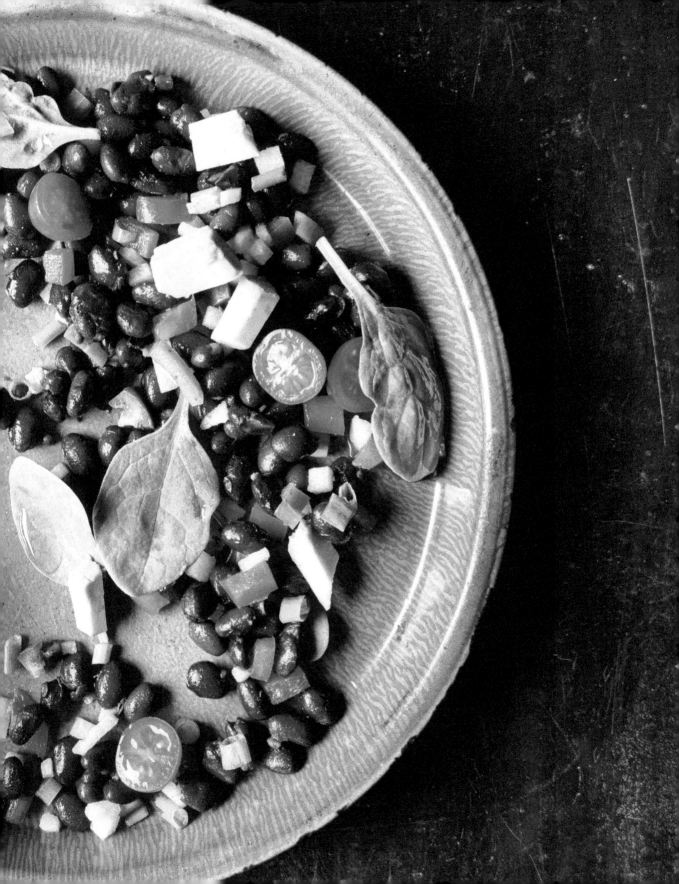

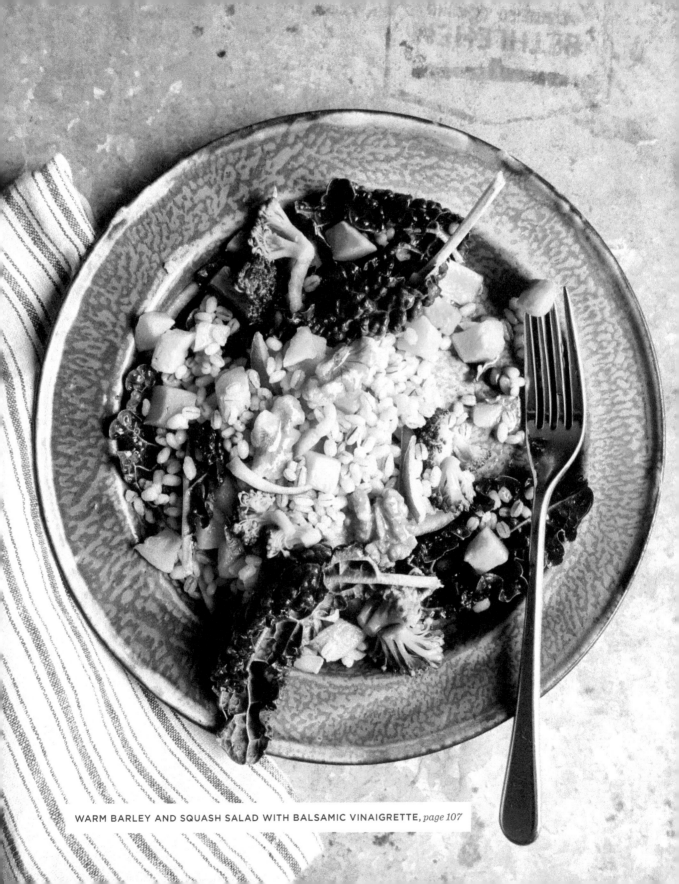

WARM BARLEY AND SQUASH SALAD WITH BALSAMIC VINAIGRETTE, *page 107*

5

Beyond Four Weeks

Congratulations on all of your amazing hard work so far! It isn't easy to get out of your normal routine, try new foods, and commit to changing the way you are eating. You've taken some incredible steps toward improving your health, and I hope you are already seeing and feeling the wonderful results. I also hope that as you have experienced the power of good nutrition and well-balanced meals, this will continue to propel your success forward so you can make this way of eating an enjoyable lifestyle—one that will add energy to your days and years to your life!

In this chapter, we are going to focus on how to make the best decisions in any situation you may find yourself in. From your favorite restaurant, to various social events, even on vacation, you can stay on track . . . while enjoying every moment!

Holidays and Social Events

I think it's important to be *very* real when it comes to special events. You can't always eat perfectly; no one does. But having a realistic plan before you get to these events will enable you to better manage your blood sugar levels. I think the old saying "Fail to plan, plan to fail" holds much truth here. Even just thinking about what food will be available at special events, how long you will be there, and what options you might have will help you form a plan.

Here are some quick tips:

Put your food on a plate. It seems so basic, I know. But you'd be surprised how many people simply hover mindlessly over the food table at events and have no idea how much they truly eat. My advice is to pick up a plate, browse the entire food table, then go back and choose a few favorites. Put them on your plate and walk away from the table to enjoy your food elsewhere while you socialize.

Serve the food in a different room. When you are in charge of the food at social events, holidays, or even just a normal weekday dinner, be sure to serve the food in a location other than the table where you are eating. (If you're at home, that means leaving all the extra food in the kitchen rather than putting it in bowls that are placed on the table.) This will give you more time to assess your hunger and fullness levels before going back for seconds.

Move after eating. Another seemingly simple strategy, but even a 10- or 15-minute walk after a meal can help prevent blood sugar levels from spiking as much as they would otherwise. This is especially helpful if you feel you may have overeaten, because it can help promote lower postmeal blood sugar levels and assist in optimal digestion.

Hydrate. Making sure that you are hydrated throughout the day is one of the easiest and most helpful ways to improve your blood sugar levels. Drinking enough water will help dilute your blood, which lowers blood sugar levels. It also helps you better assess how hungry you are, because sometimes your body mistakes thirst for hunger. Since most adults are probably not drinking enough water every day, be sure to pay attention to the color of your urine. Urine that is pale in color signifies adequate hydration. This will help every day of the year, but especially during holiday gatherings, as it will help you pay better attention to your hunger cues and prevent overeating.

Restaurants

Clients often ask about what to do when dining out, since they have less control of how food is prepared in a restaurant. So I've compiled a quick guide to strategies you can use when visiting your favorite restaurants.

CHINESE

At Chinese restaurants, added sugar is often lurking in the sauces, so be sure to request those on the side. Look for dishes based around tofu, grilled or baked proteins (make sure the protein is not breaded), and steamed veggies. Specific dishes you can ask for are cashew chicken, steamed Buddha's Feast (or Buddha's Delight), Szechwan (or Sichuan) chicken, and shrimp with broccoli.

JAPANESE

While I can't promise anything on the menu will be low in salt, there are several low-carb options available at Japanese restaurants. Look for steamed edamame and miso soup as appetizers. If you are having sushi, try hand rolls, which come without the rice, and any sashimi you like. Grilled salmon or shrimp is also usually an option, as are tuna tatami, poke with avocado and wasabi, and tofu salads. Be sure to ask your waiter if you don't see them on the menu.

INDIAN

Any type of meat or seafood kebab is a great choice at Indian restaurants. Look for korma and chicken or shrimp tandoori. Lentil- and chickpea-based dishes are also great, since these are high in fiber and protein. Just be sure they don't include rice or potatoes.

ITALIAN

While Italian food is treasured by carb lovers around the world, there are actually some really great low-carb options at any Italian restaurant. Start with caprese salad, or make a house or Italian chopped salad an entrée by adding grilled salmon, shrimp, or chicken. Look for dishes like chicken cacciatore, chicken Marsala, or chicken piccata. If you are a seafood lover, frutti di mare is also a low-carb option.

MEXICAN

You might be surprised that there are plenty of tasty low-carb options at Mexican restaurants, as well. Look for tortilla soup and request it without the extra crispy tortilla strips on top. Chicken or shrimp fajitas can also be a low-carb option if you skip the tortillas or limit yourself to one or two corn tortillas. You can also order grilled fish tacos with one or two corn tortillas, or ask to have them on a bed of lettuce. Boiled black beans are preferred to refried beans, and feel free to add low-carb toppings like salsa, pico de gallo, cilantro, guacamole, and lime juice.

DINER

One of the benefits of eating at a local diner is that these types of restaurants usually have a little bit of everything. If they serve breakfast all day, look for eggs, oatmeal, scrambles, and omelets. For lunch and dinner, look at their grilled menu and think about what combos you can make. See if you can have a grilled protein with a side salad or soup that doesn't contain any noodles or pasta. Some people prefer to order burgers and skip the bun. Whatever you decide, make the best choice possible—knowing it's a special occasion and it's likely not the same type of food as you are eating throughout the week.

On Vacation

Vacations are, of course, a time to relax, let loose, and get outside of your normal routine. While diabetes unfortunately doesn't take a day off, it's very possible to explore new foods on vacation and still maintain control of your blood sugar levels.

First of all, know that ignorance is never bliss when it comes to diabetes management. Not checking your blood sugar levels while on vacation doesn't give you any advantages. Continuing to check blood sugar levels and knowing how you're doing gives you a big advantage.

On vacation you often have more time for movement and physical activity. Whether it's walking on the beach, exploring a new city, or golfing with family, get out and enjoy the possibilities and move as much as you can.

Continue to eat at regular times. It's easy to miss meals when you are traveling, changing time zones, and outside of your normal environment. But continuing to eat meals at regularly scheduled times will help prevent unintended blood sugar fluctuations.

Pack snacks. Since delays and unexpected travel scenarios can pop up at any moment, be sure you stock up on snacks to take with you. I love nuts, individual packs of almond butter, healthy protein bars, and half a peanut butter sandwich. I also like to bring bottles of water and tea bags.

Make (some of) your own meals. If you have a small kitchen, or at least a refrigerator and microwave, you can stock up on a few staples to make yourself. Oatmeal, eggs, precut veggies, whole fruits, and nuts are all easy foods to find almost anywhere you travel, which will at least give you some basic options.

Again, your number one priority while on vacation is to have fun and enjoy a much-needed break. However, staying on track and continuing to check your blood sugar levels as best you can will provide the energy and confidence you need to know you're in control.

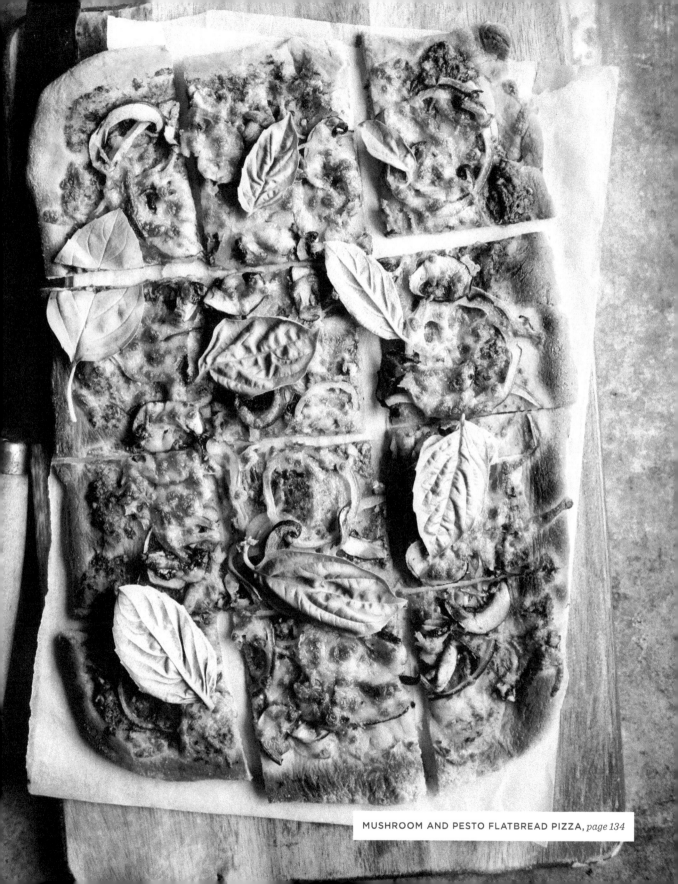

MUSHROOM AND PESTO FLATBREAD PIZZA, *page 134*

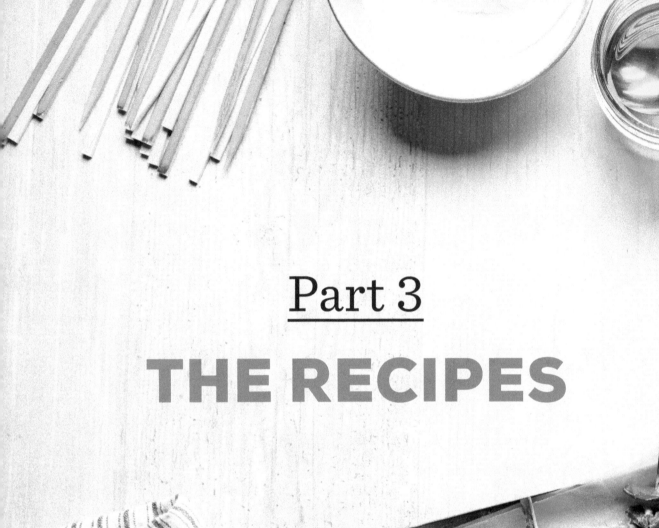

Part 3

THE RECIPES

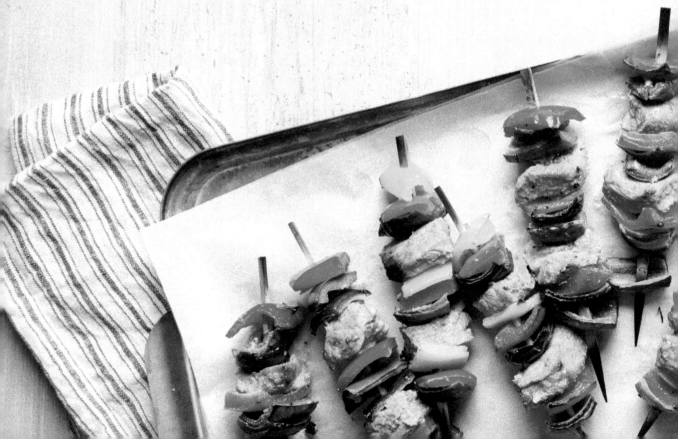

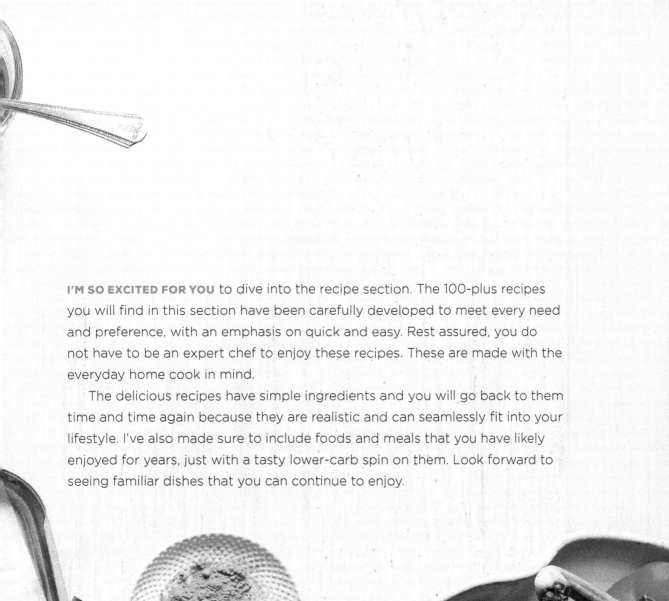

I'M SO EXCITED FOR YOU to dive into the recipe section. The 100-plus recipes you will find in this section have been carefully developed to meet every need and preference, with an emphasis on quick and easy. Rest assured, you do not have to be an expert chef to enjoy these recipes. These are made with the everyday home cook in mind.

The delicious recipes have simple ingredients and you will go back to them time and time again because they are realistic and can seamlessly fit into your lifestyle. I've also made sure to include foods and meals that you have likely enjoyed for years, just with a tasty lower-carb spin on them. Look forward to seeing familiar dishes that you can continue to enjoy.

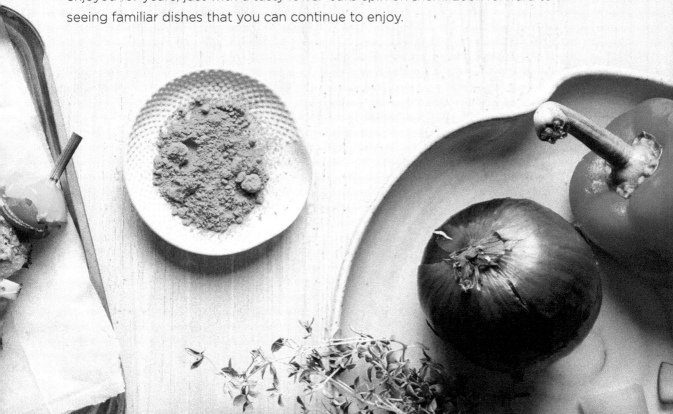

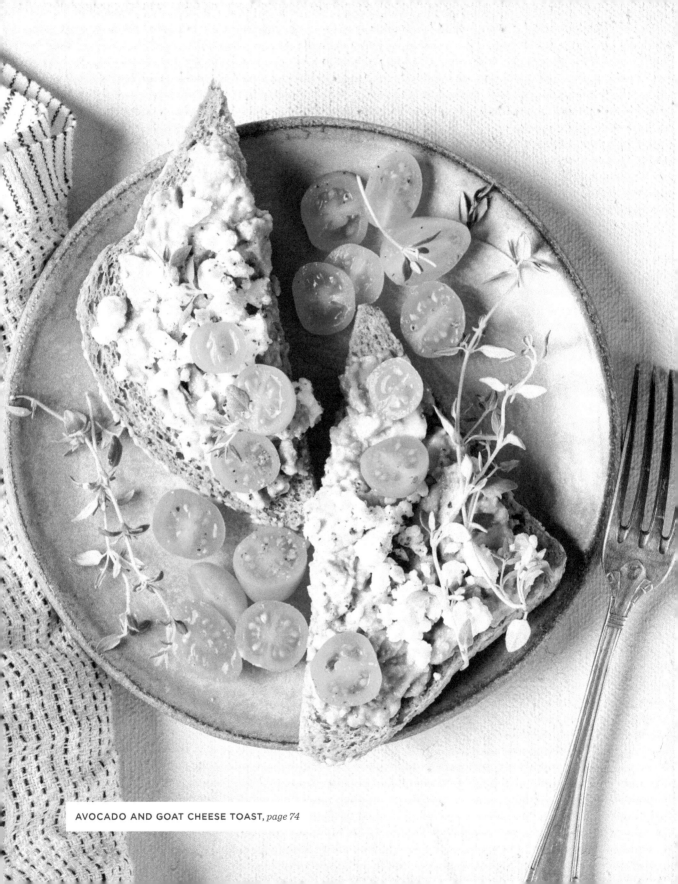

AVOCADO AND GOAT CHEESE TOAST, *page 74*

6

Breakfasts

Coconut-Berry Sunrise Smoothie

Gluten-Free | Vegetarian | Nut-Free | No-Cook | 30 Minutes or Less

I don't usually recommend smoothies because they tend to be too high in sugar, but when strategically created, they can be a great option for busy mornings. This smoothie is lower in carbs than most and super quick to make. It has the perfect blend of protein, fiber, veggies, and healthy fat, so feel free to enjoy this as a breakfast or on-the-go snack.

CARBS PER SERVING: 8g

SERVINGS: 2

PREP TIME: 5 minutes

½ cup mixed berries (blueberries, strawberries, blackberries)

1 tablespoon ground flaxseed

2 tablespoons unsweetened coconut flakes

½ cup unsweetened plain coconut milk

½ cup leafy greens (kale, spinach)

¼ cup unsweetened vanilla nonfat yogurt

½ cup ice

1. In a blender jar, combine the berries, flaxseed, coconut flakes, coconut milk, greens, yogurt, and ice.

2. Process until smooth. Serve.

Ingredient tip: Flaxseed are a great source of anti-inflammatory omega-3 fatty acids as well as dietary fiber. Be sure to choose ground flaxseed (also known as flaxseed meal) instead of whole flaxseed, since it will be easier for your body to digest and absorb their nutritional benefits.

Complete the Plate: While you can definitely eat this by itself, feel free to add 1 or 2 Breakfast Egg Bites (page 80) for extra protein and another serving of fruit or berries for a heartier, more satisfying breakfast.

PER SERVING: Calories: 181; Total Fat: 15g; Protein: 6g; Carbohydrates: 8g; Sugars: 3g; Fiber: 4g; Sodium: 24mg

Greek Yogurt Sundae

Gluten-Free | Vegetarian | No-Cook | 5-Ingredient | 30 Minutes or Less

Having a variety of quick and tasty breakfast staples makes the most important meal of the day all the easier. In this deliciously simply sundae, Greek yogurt, your choice of nuts, and ground flaxseed provide plenty of protein to get you moving, and berries and mint add sweetness and complexity to tie the quick meal together. You can prepare several sundaes on the weekend, so you have a grab-and-go breakfast every day of the week.

CARBS PER SERVING: 16g

SERVINGS: 1

PREP TIME: 5 minutes

¾ cup plain nonfat Greek yogurt

¼ cup mixed berries (blueberries, strawberries, blackberries)

2 tablespoons cashew, walnut, or almond pieces

1 tablespoon ground flaxseed

2 fresh mint leaves, shredded

1. Spoon the yogurt into a small bowl. Top with the berries, nuts, and flaxseed.

2. Garnish with the mint and serve.

Substitution tip: Use fresh or frozen berries in this sundae, as available. If using frozen, take the berries out of the freezer about 10 or 15 minutes before you make the sundae, so they can thaw.

Complete the Plate: I've never met anyone who ate too many veggies, so consider adding left-over roasted veggies, a Chocolate-Zucchini Muffin (page 76), or a serving of Brussels Sprout Hash and Eggs (page 84), or top with Oat and Walnut Granola (page 75).

PER SERVING: Calories: 237; Total Fat: 11g; Protein: 21g; Carbohydrates: 16g; Sugars: 9g; Fiber: 4g; Sodium: 64mg

Avocado and Goat Cheese Toast

Vegetarian | Nut-Free | No-Cook | 5-Ingredient | 30 Minutes or Less

Sometimes the simplest of breakfasts can be the most filling and delicious. Loaded with healthy fats and plenty of savory flavor, this quick, no-frills breakfast can be ready in the amount of time it takes to toast your bread. If you want a little something more, sprinkle on some crushed red pepper flakes, or add 2 tablespoons of pomegranate seeds or 2 slices of crumbled bacon for even more flavor and flair.

CARBS PER SERVING: 18g
SERVINGS: 2 (1 slice each)
PREP TIME: 5 minutes

2 slices whole-wheat thin-sliced bread (I love Ezekiel sprouted bread and Dave's Killer Bread)

½ avocado

2 tablespoons crumbled goat cheese

Salt

1. In a toaster or broiler, toast the bread until browned.

2. Remove the flesh from the avocado. In a medium bowl, use a fork to mash the avocado flesh. Spread it onto the toast.

3. Sprinkle with the goat cheese and season lightly with salt.

4. Add any toppings and serve.

Option tip: The options for topping avocado toast are endless. Some more ideas include adding a handful of microgreens, a tablespoon of crushed nuts, a tablespoon of Parmesan cheese, a couple of tomato slices, or a poached egg. Just remember that any add-ins will change the nutrient profile.

Complete the Plate: I definitely recommend adding an extra protein source to this meal. Great additions would be a Greek Yogurt Sundae (page 73), Breakfast Egg Bites (page 80), or Homemade Turkey Breakfast Sausage (page 86).

PER SERVING: Calories: 137; Total Fat: 6g; Protein: 5g; Carbohydrates: 18g; Sugars: 0g; Fiber: 5g; Sodium: 195mg

Oat and Walnut Granola

Gluten-Free | Vegan

Granola is a great way to start the day, but most commercial brands have eye-opening amounts of sugar. This version is lightly sweet from the naturally sweet applesauce and dried cherries but has no added sugar, making it a healthier alternative to store-bought. Be sure to let it sit undisturbed after cooking, as this is the secret to creating the clumps in your finished granola.

CARBS PER SERVING: 20g
SERVINGS: 16 (⅓ cup each)
PREP TIME: 10 minutes
COOK TIME: 30 minutes

4 cups rolled oats

1 cup walnut pieces

½ cup pepitas

¼ teaspoon salt

1 teaspoon ground cinnamon

1 teaspoon ground ginger

½ cup coconut oil, melted

½ cup unsweetened applesauce

1 teaspoon vanilla extract

½ cup dried cherries

1. Preheat the oven to 350°F. Line a baking sheet with parchment paper.

2. In a large bowl, toss the oats, walnuts, pepitas, salt, cinnamon, and ginger.

3. In a large measuring cup, combine the coconut oil, applesauce, and vanilla. Pour over the dry mixture and mix well.

4. Transfer the mixture to the prepared baking sheet. Cook for 30 minutes, stirring about halfway through. Remove from the oven and let the granola sit undisturbed until completely cool. Break the granola into pieces, and stir in the dried cherries.

5. Transfer to an airtight container, and store at room temperature for up to 2 weeks.

Option tip: For a higher-protein granola, mix in up to ½ cup hemp seeds or flaxseed after cooking, along with the cherries.

Complete the Plate: This granola is the perfect way to top a Greek Yogurt Sundae (page 73) to make it a filling and complete meal.

PER SERVING: Calories: 224; Total Fat: 15g; Protein: 5g; Carbohydrates: 20g; Sugars: 5g; Fiber: 3g; Sodium: 30mg

Chocolate-Zucchini Muffins

Gluten-Free | Vegetarian | Nut-Free

Zucchini takes on any flavor you mix it with, making it a great vegetable to incorporate into your breakfast. You might not even know it's there if you didn't make these muffins yourself. Summer squash, such as zucchini, may not be loaded with as many nutrients as other vegetables, but it does contain carotenes and has some anticancer benefits, making it a great addition to your diet.

CARBS PER SERVING: 16g
SERVINGS: 12
(1 muffin each)
PREP TIME: 15 minutes
COOK TIME: 20 minutes

1½ cups grated zucchini

1½ cups rolled oats

1 teaspoon ground cinnamon

2 teaspoons baking powder

¼ teaspoon salt

1 large egg

1 teaspoon vanilla extract

¼ cup coconut oil, melted

½ cup unsweetened applesauce

¼ cup honey

¼ cup dark chocolate chips

1. Preheat the oven to 350°F. Grease the cups of a 12-cup muffin tin or line with paper baking liners. Set aside.

2. Place the zucchini in a colander over the sink to drain.

3. In a blender jar, process the oats until they resemble flour. Transfer to a medium mixing bowl and add the cinnamon, baking powder, and salt. Mix well.

4. In another large mixing bowl, combine the egg, vanilla, coconut oil, applesauce, and honey. Stir to combine.

5. Press the zucchini into the colander, draining any liquids, and add to the wet mixture.

6. Stir the dry mixture into the wet mixture, and mix until no dry spots remain. Fold in the chocolate chips.

7. Transfer the batter to the muffin tin, filling each cup a little over halfway. Cook for 16 to 18 minutes until the muffins are lightly browned and a toothpick inserted in the center comes out clean.

8. Store in an airtight container, refrigerated, for up to 5 days.

Option tip: Add more protein to the muffins by adding ½ cup walnut pieces along with the chocolate chips. If you make more muffins than you need, you can freeze them for up to 3 months to ensure you have a quick, healthy breakfast or snack for any day of the week.

 Complete the Plate: Feel free to have one or two of these muffins for your breakfast with an additional protein. They are great with Brussels Sprout Hash and Eggs (page 84); Spinach, Artichoke, and Goat Cheese Breakfast Bake (page 85); or simply a serving of Greek yogurt.

PER SERVING: Calories: 121; Total Fat: 7g; Protein: 2g; Carbohydrates: 16g; Sugars: 7g; Fiber: 2g; Sodium: 106mg

Gluten-Free Carrot and Oat Pancakes

Gluten-Free | Vegetarian | 30 Minutes or Less

Traditional pancake mixes often contain sneaky added sugars and trans fats, but these gluten-free, veggie-rich pancakes are perfect for every day. Using eggs, cottage cheese, and almond milk, these flavorful flapjacks are protein rich and taste every bit as good as more traditional versions. Top them with maple syrup–sweetened Greek yogurt for a healthier, more blood-sugar-stabilizing option than syrup alone.

CARBS PER SERVING: 24g

SERVINGS: 4

(3 pancakes each)

PREP TIME: 10 minutes

COOK TIME: 20 minutes

1 cup rolled oats

1 cup shredded carrots

1 cup low-fat cottage cheese

2 eggs

½ cup unsweetened plain almond milk

1 teaspoon baking powder

½ teaspoon ground cinnamon

2 tablespoons ground flaxseed

¼ cup plain nonfat Greek yogurt

1 tablespoon pure maple syrup

2 teaspoons canola oil, divided

1. In a blender jar, process the oats until they resemble flour. Add the carrots, cottage cheese, eggs, almond milk, baking powder, cinnamon, and flaxseed to the jar. Process until smooth.

2. In a small bowl, combine the yogurt and maple syrup and stir well. Set aside.

3. In a large skillet, heat 1 teaspoon of oil over medium heat. Using a measuring cup, add ¼ cup of batter per pancake to the skillet. Cook for 1 to 2 minutes until bubbles form on the surface, and flip the pancakes. Cook for another minute until the pancakes are browned and cooked through. Repeat with the remaining 1 teaspoon of oil and remaining batter.

4. Serve warm topped with the maple yogurt.

Ingredient tip: While oats are naturally gluten free, many brands are processed in facilities that also process grains with gluten, making cross-contamination risk high. If you are sensitive to gluten, be sure to select oats that are labeled as gluten free.

 Complete the Plate: This meal will check every nutrient box, but you can always add a side of Homemade Turkey Breakfast Sausage (page 86) or pair with the Coconut-Berry Sunrise Smoothie (page 72).

PER SERVING: Calories: 226; Total Fat: 8g; Protein: 15g; Carbohydrates: 24g; Sugars: 7g; Fiber: 4g; Sodium: 403mg

Breakfast Egg Bites

Gluten-Free : Vegetarian

Having savory breakfast staples on hand is perfect for busy mornings, and these are just the thing to stock up on. They can be made in advance, so whip up a batch on the weekend and enjoy them throughout the week for a quick breakfast that you don't have to turn your stove on for.

CARBS PER SERVING: 3g

SERVINGS: 8

(1 egg bite each)

PREP TIME: 10 minutes

COOK TIME: 25 minutes

Nonstick cooking spray

6 eggs, beaten

¼ cup unsweetened plain almond milk

1 red bell pepper, diced

1 cup chopped spinach

¼ cup crumbled goat cheese

½ cup sliced brown mushrooms

¼ cup sliced sun-dried tomatoes

Salt

Freshly ground black pepper

1. Preheat the oven to 350°F. Spray 8 muffin cups of a 12-cup muffin tin with nonstick cooking spray. Set aside.

2. In a large mixing bowl, combine the eggs, almond milk, bell pepper, spinach, goat cheese, mushrooms, and tomatoes. Season with salt and pepper.

3. Fill the prepared muffin cups three-fourths full with the egg mixture. Bake for 20 to 25 minutes until the eggs are set. Let cool slightly and remove the egg bites from the muffin tin.

4. Serve warm, or store in an airtight container in the refrigerator for up to 5 days or in the freezer for up to 1 month.

Technique tip: For a busy morning, you can make these egg bites in single servings in the microwave. Spray a microwave-safe mug with nonstick cooking spray and add 1 beaten egg, along with 1 tablespoon unsweetened plain almond milk, 1 tablespoon minced bell pepper, a couple of tablespoons chopped spinach, and a few mushroom and sun-dried tomato slices. Season with a pinch salt and pepper. Microwave on high for 1½ to 2 minutes until the eggs begin to set.

 Complete the Plate: You will want to add some healthy carbs to this meal. Consider Chocolate-Zucchini Muffins (page 76), Gluten-Free Carrot and Oat Pancakes (page 78), Oat and Walnut Granola (page 75), or simply a serving of your favorite fruit.

PER SERVING: Calories: 67; Total Fat: 4g; Protein: 6g; Carbohydrates: 3g; Sugars: 2g; Fiber: 1g; Sodium: 127mg

Crispy Breakfast Pita with Egg and Canadian Bacon

Nut-Free | 30 Minutes or Less

Even on the weekends when you have a little more time for breakfast, this is a quick fix that will get your day started off right. Topped with a pile of flavorful and nutrient-dense microgreens, this is a simple meal that you will go back to again and again. This has become a favorite go-to breakfast meal for my husband and me since it is perfectly balanced and keeps us full for hours.

CARBS PER SERVING: 20g
SERVINGS: 2
PREP TIME: 5 minutes
COOK TIME: 15 minutes

1 (6-inch) whole-grain pita bread

3 teaspoons extra-virgin olive oil, divided

2 eggs

2 Canadian bacon slices

Juice of ½ lemon

1 cup microgreens

2 tablespoons crumbled goat cheese

Freshly ground black pepper

1. Heat a large skillet over medium heat. Cut the pita bread in half and brush each side of both halves with ¼ teaspoon of olive oil (using a total of 1 teaspoon oil). Cook for 2 to 3 minutes on each side, then remove from the skillet.

2. In the same skillet, heat 1 teaspoon of oil over medium heat. Crack the eggs into the skillet and cook until the eggs are set, 2 to 3 minutes. Remove from the skillet.

3. In the same skillet, cook the Canadian bacon for 3 to 5 minutes, flipping once.

4. In a large bowl, whisk together the remaining 1 teaspoon of oil and the lemon juice. Add the microgreens and toss to combine.

5. Top each pita half with half of the microgreens, 1 piece of bacon, 1 egg, and 1 tablespoon of goat cheese. Season with pepper and serve.

Ingredient tip: Microgreens are the immature edible greens of any number of vegetables. They are easy to grow yourself or can be found at farmers' markets and specialty and natural grocers year-round. There are many different varieties and you can play around and see which you prefer. If you can't find microgreens, feel free to substitute arugula, baby kale, spinach, or any other leafy green you like.

 Complete the Plate: This is a complete meal in itself, but you can always add a healthy fat by topping it with some fresh avocado slices or guacamole. And feel free to add an extra egg or slice of Canadian bacon for a protein boost.

PER SERVING: Calories: 250; Total Fat: 14g; Protein: 13g; Carbohydrates: 20g; Sugars: 1g; Fiber: 3g; Sodium: 398mg

Brussels Sprout Hash and Eggs

Gluten-Free | Vegetarian | Dairy-Free | Nut-Free | 5-Ingredient | 30 Minutes or Less

When cooked at the peak of freshness, Brussels sprouts need little to enhance their subtle sweetness. In this easy hash preparation, lemon and garlic provide plenty of well-balanced flavor. The hash reheats well, so feel free to make a double batch to enjoy throughout the week.

CARBS PER SERVING: 12g
SERVINGS: 4
PREP TIME: 15 minutes
COOK TIME: 15 minutes

3 teaspoons extra-virgin olive oil, divided

1 pound Brussels sprouts, sliced

2 garlic cloves, thinly sliced

¼ teaspoon salt

Juice of 1 lemon

4 eggs

1. In a large skillet, heat 1½ teaspoons of oil over medium heat. Add the Brussels sprouts and toss. Cook, stirring regularly, for 6 to 8 minutes until browned and softened. Add the garlic and continue to cook until fragrant, about 1 minute. Season with the salt and lemon juice. Transfer to a serving dish.

2. In the same pan, heat the remaining 1½ teaspoons of oil over medium-high heat. Crack the eggs into the pan. Fry for 2 to 4 minutes, flip, and continue cooking to desired doneness. Serve over the bed of hash.

Make-ahead tip: Brussels sprouts, like other brassica vegetables, are easy to prep in advance and hold up well both raw and cooked. Prep the Brussels sprouts up to 5 days in advance by slicing them when you have a free moment. Refrigerate in an airtight container until ready for use.

 Complete the Plate: This meal is very low in carbs, so it is a good option for days you wake up and your blood sugar is higher than desired. But you can also add an additional serving of carbs and protein, such as Crispy Breakfast Pita with Egg and Canadian Bacon (page 82) or Gluten-Free Carrot and Oat Pancakes (page 78).

PER SERVING: Calories: 158; Total Fat: 9g; Protein: 10g; Carbohydrates: 12g; Sugars: 4g; Fiber: 4g; Sodium: 234mg

Spinach, Artichoke, and Goat Cheese Breakfast Bake

Gluten-Free | Vegetarian

Breakfast bakes that are prepared, cooked, and served in one dish are one of my favorite time-saving strategies, especially as the mom of a toddler. And since this recipe makes 8 servings, you can enjoy this one throughout the week for easier mornings. Artichokes are one of the highest-fiber vegetables and loaded with inulin, a specific type of prebiotic fiber that has proven helpful in controlling blood sugar levels. Enjoy!

CARBS PER SERVING: 6g

SERVINGS: 8

PREP TIME: 10 minutes

COOK TIME: 35 minutes

Nonstick cooking spray

1 (10-ounce) package frozen spinach, thawed and drained

1 (14-ounce) can artichoke hearts, drained

¼ cup finely chopped red bell pepper

2 garlic cloves, minced

8 eggs, lightly beaten

¼ cup unsweetened plain almond milk

½ teaspoon salt

½ teaspoon freshly ground black pepper

½ cup crumbled goat cheese

1. Preheat the oven to 375°F. Spray an 8-by-8-inch baking dish with nonstick cooking spray.

2. In a large mixing bowl, combine the spinach, artichoke hearts, bell pepper, garlic, eggs, almond milk, salt, and pepper. Stir well to combine.

3. Transfer the mixture to the baking dish. Sprinkle with the goat cheese.

4. Bake for 35 minutes until the eggs are set. Serve warm.

Option tip: Spice things up for breakfast by adding a scant teaspoon of red pepper flakes to this dish.

 Complete the Plate: This is a very-low-carb yet high-protein breakfast, so feel free to have 2 or 3 servings, along with a Chocolate-Zucchini Muffin (page 76), if desired. Or you could simply have it with a cup of your favorite berries or a small baked sweet potato.

PER SERVING: Calories: 104; Total Fat: 5g; Protein: 9g; Carbohydrates: 6g; Sugars: 1g; Fiber: 2g; Sodium: 488mg

Homemade Turkey Breakfast Sausage

Gluten-Free | Nut-Free | 5-Ingredient | 30 Minutes or Less

It may have never crossed your mind to make your own sausage at home, but it is much easier than you might think. This breakfast sausage can be made with some common spices you may already have in your cupboard. You will be impressed with just how simple it is to replicate the flavor of the store-bought versions, only without the unwanted and hidden sugar and salt.

CARBS PER SERVING: 0g
SERVINGS: 8 (1 patty each)
PREP TIME: 10 minutes
COOK TIME: 10 minutes

1 pound lean ground turkey

½ teaspoon salt

½ teaspoon dried sage

½ teaspoon dried thyme

½ teaspoon freshly ground black pepper

¼ teaspoon ground fennel seeds

1 teaspoon extra-virgin olive oil

1. In a large mixing bowl, combine the ground turkey, salt, sage, thyme, pepper, and fennel. Mix well.

2. Shape the meat into 8 small, round patties.

3. Heat the olive oil in a skillet over medium-high heat. Cook the patties in the skillet for 3 to 4 minutes on each side until browned and cooked through.

4. Serve warm, or store in an airtight container in the refrigerator for up to 3 days or in the freezer for up to 1 month.

Technique tip: If you are using the turkey sausage for Sweet Potato, Onion, and Turkey Sausage Hash (page 87), skip steps 2 and 3, and add the bulk sausage to the pan as is when called for in the recipe.

Complete the Plate: While this is a great source of protein, you will want to add more to complete this breakfast. The easiest complete meal would be to make Sweet Potato, Onion, and Turkey Sausage Hash (page 87), but I also love to serve these with Gluten-Free Carrot and Oat Pancakes (page 78) for a nice weekend brunch.

PER SERVING: Calories: 92; Total Fat: 5g; Protein: 11g; Carbohydrates: 0g; Sugars: 0g; Fiber: 0g; Sodium: 156mg

Sweet Potato, Onion, and Turkey Sausage Hash

Gluten-Free | Nut-Free

Sweet potatoes are higher in fiber (even more so when they're not peeled, as in this dish) than white potatoes, making them a better option for controlling your blood sugar levels. They are also a great source of vitamin A, which may improve the function of your pancreatic beta cells—the cells that produce, store, and release insulin. Serve this hash with a poached or hard-boiled egg on top for an even more filling breakfast.

CARBS PER SERVING: 16g

SERVINGS: 4

PREP TIME: 10 minutes

COOK TIME: 25 minutes

1 tablespoon extra-virgin oil

2 medium sweet potatoes, cut into ½-inch dice

½ recipe Homemade Turkey Breakfast Sausage (page 86)

1 small onion, chopped

½ red bell pepper, seeded and chopped

2 garlic cloves, minced

Chopped fresh parsley, for garnish

1. In a large skillet, heat the oil over medium-high heat. Add the sweet potatoes and cook, stirring occasionally, for 12 to 15 minutes until they brown and begin to soften.

2. Add the turkey sausage in bulk, onion, bell pepper, and garlic. Cook for 5 to 6 minutes until the turkey sausage is cooked through and the vegetables soften.

3. Garnish with parsley and serve warm.

Ingredient tip: Sweet potatoes are lower than white potatoes on the glycemic index, which ranks carb-containing foods by how much they can affect your blood sugar levels. Foods with a greater number are usually processed or contain added sugars, while those with a smaller number are more slowly digested and metabolized and cause a lower and slower rise in your blood sugar levels.

Complete the Plate: While this recipe includes veggies, protein, and carbs, it's a good idea to add a bit more to ensure you are satisfied until your next meal. You can double the portion of Homemade Turkey Breakfast Sausage (page 86) or serve with Spinach, Artichoke, and Goat Cheese Breakfast Bake (page 85).

PER SERVING: Calories: 190; Total Fat: 9g; Protein: 12g; Carbohydrates: 16g; Sugars: 7g; Fiber: 3g; Sodium: 197mg

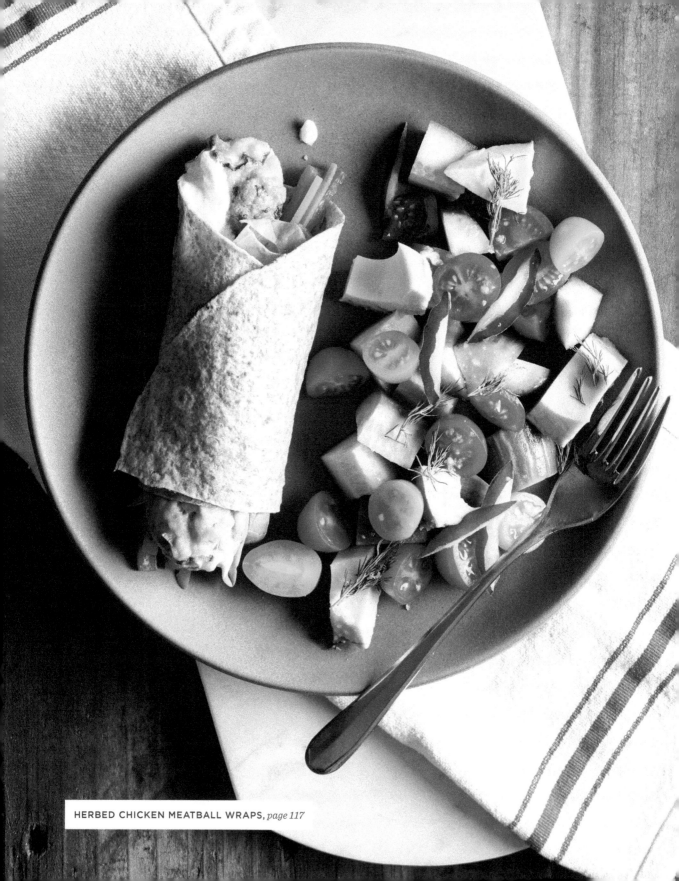

HERBED CHICKEN MEATBALL WRAPS, *page 117*

7

Soups, Salads, and Sandwiches

Gazpacho

Gluten-Free | Vegetarian | Dairy-Free | Nut-Free | No-Cook | 30 Minutes or Less

Gazpacho is a wonderful soup for a warm day. Cool and refreshing, the tomato-based soup is fresh and requires no cooking. Prepare it at least an hour before serving to allow the flavors to blend together into a flavorful, veggie-forward powerhouse.

CARBS PER SERVING: 24g
SERVINGS: 4
PREP TIME: 15 minutes

3 pounds ripe tomatoes, chopped

1 cup low-sodium tomato juice

½ red onion, chopped

1 cucumber, peeled, seeded, and chopped

1 red bell pepper, seeded and chopped

2 celery stalks, chopped

2 tablespoons chopped fresh parsley

2 garlic cloves, chopped

2 tablespoons extra-virgin olive oil

2 tablespoons red wine vinegar

1 teaspoon honey

½ teaspoon salt

¼ teaspoon freshly ground black pepper

1. In a blender jar, combine the tomatoes, tomato juice, onion, cucumber, bell pepper, celery, parsley, garlic, olive oil, vinegar, honey, salt, and pepper. Pulse until blended but still slightly chunky.

2. Adjust the seasonings as needed and serve.

3. To store, transfer to a nonreactive, airtight container and refrigerate for up to 3 days.

Option tip: For a little kick in the soup, add a seeded jalapeño or serrano pepper when blending.

 Complete the Plate: This is a great addition to any meal. Complete the plate by adding a side of your favorite lean protein and roasted veggies or a hearty salad like Blueberry and Chicken Salad on a Bed of Greens (page 110).

PER SERVING: Calories: 170; Total Fat: 8g; Protein: 5g; Carbohydrates: 24g; Sugars: 16g; Fiber: 6g; Sodium: 332mg

Tomato and Kale Soup

Gluten-Free | Vegan | Dairy-Free | Nut-Free | 30 Minutes or Less

Baby kale is a mild, leafy green that gives this soup a boost of vitamin power. Loaded with beta-carotene, vitamins A and C, and chlorophyll, kale is an excellent addition to soups, where its sturdy leaves hold up well to cooking. This simple Italian-flavored soup is a perfect complement to sandwiches and salads.

CARBS PER SERVING: 31g

SERVINGS: 4

PREP TIME: 10 minutes

COOK TIME: 15 minutes

1 tablespoon extra-virgin olive oil

1 medium onion, chopped

2 carrots, finely chopped

3 garlic cloves, minced

4 cups low-sodium vegetable broth

1 (28-ounce) can crushed tomatoes

½ teaspoon dried oregano

¼ teaspoon dried basil

4 cups chopped baby kale leaves

¼ teaspoon salt

1. In a large pot, heat the oil over medium heat. Add the onion and carrots to the pan. Sauté for 3 to 5 minutes until they begin to soften. Add the garlic and sauté for 30 seconds more, until fragrant.

2. Add the vegetable broth, tomatoes, oregano, and basil to the pot and bring to a boil. Reduce the heat to low and simmer for 5 minutes.

3. Using an immersion blender, purée the soup.

4. Add the kale and simmer for 3 more minutes. Season with the salt. Serve immediately.

Ingredient tip: Kale is available year-round but is at its peak in the cooler months. To save on prep time, you can also buy bags of prewashed cut and cleaned kale to add to soups, salads, omelets, and other cooked dishes like this one.

 Complete the Plate: Add your favorite grilled or baked lean protein, or the Turkey Meatloaf Muffins (page 165) or the Peppercorn-Crusted Baked Salmon (page 193).

PER SERVING: Calories: 170; Total Fat: 5g; Protein: 6g; Carbohydrates: 31g; Sugars: 13g; Fiber: 9g; Sodium: 600mg

Comforting Summer Squash Soup with Crispy Chickpeas

Gluten-Free | Vegetarian | Nut-Free | 30 Minutes or Less

Everyone needs an easy, nourishing soup made with simple ingredients that are always on hand. Since this takes only 30 minutes to make, it's a great choice for those days when you are feeling a little under the weather. This hydrating soup contains a good source of electrolytes (sodium, potassium, and calcium), so sip away while fueling your body!

CARBS PER SERVING: 24g

SERVINGS: 4

PREP TIME: 10 minutes

COOK TIME: 20 minutes

1 (15-ounce) can low-sodium chickpeas, drained and rinsed

1 teaspoon extra-virgin olive oil, plus 1 tablespoon

¼ teaspoon smoked paprika

Pinch salt, plus ½ teaspoon

3 medium zucchini, coarsely chopped

3 cups low-sodium vegetable broth

½ onion, diced

3 garlic cloves, minced

2 tablespoons plain low-fat Greek yogurt

Freshly ground black pepper

1. Preheat the oven to 425°F. Line a baking sheet with parchment paper.

2. In a medium mixing bowl, toss the chickpeas with 1 teaspoon of olive oil, the smoked paprika, and a pinch salt. Transfer to the prepared baking sheet and roast until crispy, about 20 minutes, stirring once. Set aside.

3. Meanwhile, in a medium pot, heat the remaining 1 tablespoon of oil over medium heat.

4. Add the zucchini, broth, onion, and garlic to the pot, and bring to a boil. Reduce the heat to a simmer, and cook until the zucchini and onion are tender, about 20 minutes.

5. In a blender jar, or using an immersion blender, purée the soup. Return to the pot.

6. Add the yogurt, remaining ½ teaspoon of salt, and pepper, and stir well. Serve topped with the roasted chickpeas.

Substitution tip: Try other summer squash instead of zucchini. Great choices are yellow zucchini or yellow squash.

 Complete the Plate: While this recipe completes the plate, it is still low in energy (aka calories), so it's a good idea to add more. I recommend another protein, like Easy Chicken Cacciatore (page 160), and another vegetable dish, like Roasted Lemon and Garlic Broccoli (page 122).

PER SERVING: Calories: 188; Total Fat: 7g; Protein: 8g; Carbohydrates: 24g; Sugars: 7g; Fiber: 7g; Sodium: 528mg

Curried Carrot Soup

Gluten-Free | Vegan | Dairy-Free | Nut-Free | 30 Minutes or Less | Instant Pot Easy

If you are looking for new ways to add more veggies to your meals, this is a great way to start. Curry powder contains turmeric, which has been found to have powerful components called curcumin that have the potential to prevent chronic diseases such as arthritis, cancer, heart disease, and Alzheimer's disease, according to *The American Dietetic Association Complete Food and Nutrition Guide*.

CARBS PER SERVING: 13g
SERVINGS: 6
PREP TIME: 10 minutes
COOK TIME: 5 minutes

1 tablespoon extra-virgin olive oil

1 small onion, coarsely chopped

2 celery stalks, coarsely chopped

1½ teaspoons curry powder

1 teaspoon ground cumin

1 teaspoon minced fresh ginger

6 medium carrots, roughly chopped

4 cups low-sodium vegetable broth

¼ teaspoon salt

1 cup canned coconut milk

¼ teaspoon freshly ground black pepper

1 tablespoon chopped fresh cilantro

1. Heat an Instant Pot to high and add the olive oil.

2. Sauté the onion and celery for 2 to 3 minutes. Add the curry powder, cumin, and ginger to the pot and cook until fragrant, about 30 seconds.

3. Add the carrots, vegetable broth, and salt to the pot. Close and seal, and set for 5 minutes on high. Allow the pressure to release naturally.

4. In a blender jar, carefully purée the soup in batches and transfer back to the pot.

5. Stir in the coconut milk and pepper, and heat through. Top with the cilantro and serve.

Option tip: If you don't have an Instant Pot, make this soup on the stove following the same instructions, but in step 3, bring the soup to a simmer and cook for 15 minutes until the carrots are tender. Purée and finish the soup as instructed.

 Complete the Plate: This soup is low in protein and carbs. Pair with Tuna, Hummus, and Veggie Wraps (page 115) or Salmon, Quinoa, and Avocado Salad (page 111).

PER SERVING: Calories: 145; Total Fat: 11g; Protein: 2g; Carbohydrates: 13g; Sugars: 4g; Fiber: 3g; Sodium: 238mg

Thai Peanut, Carrot, and Shrimp Soup

Gluten-Free | Dairy-Free | 30 Minutes or Less

Using carrots, peanuts, and almond milk to form a rich yet dairy-free base, this simple Thai-inspired soup pairs really well with Winter Chicken and Citrus Salad (page 109). Use easy-peel shrimp to make prep even quicker and have the soup ready in only 20 minutes. Or omit the shrimp for a vegan version of this dish.

CARBS PER SERVING: 17g
SERVINGS: 4
PREP TIME: 10 minutes
COOK TIME: 10 minutes

- 1 tablespoon coconut oil
- 1 tablespoon Thai red curry paste
- ½ onion, sliced
- 3 garlic cloves, minced
- 2 cups chopped carrots
- ½ cup whole unsalted peanuts
- 4 cups low-sodium vegetable broth
- ½ cup unsweetened plain almond milk
- ½ pound shrimp, peeled and deveined
- Minced fresh cilantro, for garnish

1. In a large pan, heat the oil over medium-high heat until shimmering.
2. Add the curry paste and cook, stirring constantly, for 1 minute. Add the onion, garlic, carrots, and peanuts to the pan, and continue to cook for 2 to 3 minutes until the onion begins to soften.
3. Add the broth and bring to a boil. Reduce the heat to low and simmer for 5 to 6 minutes until the carrots are tender.
4. Using an immersion blender or in a blender, purée the soup until smooth and return it to the pot. With the heat still on low, add the almond milk and stir to combine. Add the shrimp to the pot and cook for 2 to 3 minutes until cooked through.
5. Garnish with cilantro and serve.

Thai Peanut, Carrot, and Shrimp Soup, *continued*

Ingredient tip: Thai red curry paste is a thick paste traditionally made with red chiles, dry spices, freshly ground herbs, garlic, and a few other flavorful, fresh ingredients. Despite the chiles, it isn't too spicy, so it provides a perfectly balanced taste. Find it in the Asian foods aisle of your supermarket or in an Asian grocery or health food store.

 Complete the Plate: This flavorful soup has about 2 ounces of protein per serving, so you might want to add another carb-and-protein serving like a Red Pepper, Goat Cheese, and Arugula Open-Faced Grilled Sandwich (page 113).

PER SERVING: Calories: 237; Total Fat: 14g; Protein: 14g; Carbohydrates: 17g; Sugars: 6g; Fiber: 5g; Sodium: 619mg

Chicken Tortilla Soup

Gluten-Free | Nut-Free

Tortilla soup is a delicious favorite that can be made healthier by baking the tortilla strips instead of the usual frying, without missing out on any of the flavor. Using boneless, skinless chicken breasts, this is a low-fat soup that pairs well with many salads for a filling meal with little work.

CARBS PER SERVING: 13g
SERVINGS: 4
PREP TIME: 10 minutes
COOK TIME: 35 minutes

1 tablespoon extra-virgin olive oil

1 onion, thinly sliced

1 garlic clove, minced

1 jalapeño pepper, diced

2 boneless, skinless chicken breasts

4 cups low-sodium chicken broth

1 roma tomato, diced

½ teaspoon salt

2 (6-inch) corn tortillas, cut into thin strips

Nonstick cooking spray

Juice of 1 lime

Minced fresh cilantro, for garnish

¼ cup shredded cheddar cheese, for garnish

1. In a medium pot, heat the oil over medium-high heat. Add the onion and cook for 3 to 5 minutes until it begins to soften. Add the garlic and jalapeño, and cook until fragrant, about 1 minute more.

2. Add the chicken, chicken broth, tomato, and salt to the pot and bring to a boil. Reduce the heat to medium and simmer gently for 20 to 25 minutes until the chicken breasts are cooked through. Remove the chicken from the pot and set aside.

3. Preheat a broiler to high.

4. Spray the tortilla strips with nonstick cooking spray and toss to coat. Spread in a single layer on a baking sheet and broil for 3 to 5 minutes, flipping once, until crisp.

5. When the chicken is cool enough to handle, shred it with two forks and return to the pot.

6. Season the soup with the lime juice. Serve hot, garnished with cilantro, cheese, and tortilla strips.

◆➤

Option tip: Add several cubes of avocado along with the cheese as a garnish.

 Complete the Plate: Create an entire Mexican-inspired meal by adding Spicy Roasted Cauliflower with Lime (page 124) and Black Bean Enchilada Skillet Casserole (page 135).

PER SERVING: Calories: 191; Total Fat: 8g; Protein: 19g; Carbohydrates: 13g; Sugars: 2g; Fiber: 2g; Sodium: 482mg

Beef and Mushroom Barley Soup

Dairy-Free | Nut-Free | Slow Cooker Easy | Instant Pot Easy

Beef and mushroom barley soup is comfort food at its best, and this classic recipe delivers all of the flavor in just a fraction of the time as the long-simmered original. Make this soup in an Instant Pot and you will have tender, falling-apart stew meat in just over an hour of cooking time. If you don't have an Instant Pot, a slow cooker will work just as well. Brown the meat and vegetables in a pan in the same order as the recipe, and transfer it all to the slow cooker along with the broth and water. Set the slow cooker to high for 3 hours or low for 6 hours. Then add the barley and cook for an additional 1 hour.

CARBS PER SERVING: 19g

SERVINGS: 6

PREP TIME: 10 minutes

COOK TIME: 1 hour, 20 minutes

1 pound beef stew meat, cubed

¼ teaspoon salt

¼ teaspoon freshly ground black pepper

1 tablespoon extra-virgin olive oil

8 ounces sliced mushrooms

1 onion, chopped

2 carrots, chopped

3 celery stalks, chopped

6 garlic cloves, minced

½ teaspoon dried thyme

4 cups low-sodium beef broth

1 cup water

½ cup pearl barley

1. Season the meat with the salt and pepper.

2. In an Instant Pot, heat the oil over high heat. Add the meat and brown on all sides. Remove the meat from the pot and set aside.

3. Add the mushrooms to the pot and cook for 1 to 2 minutes, until they begin to soften. Remove the mushrooms and set aside with the meat.

4. Add the onion, carrots, and celery to the pot. Sauté for 3 to 4 minutes until the vegetables begin to soften. Add the garlic and continue to cook until fragrant, about 30 seconds longer.

5. Return the meat and mushrooms to the pot, then add the thyme, beef broth, and water. Set the pressure to high and cook for 15 minutes. Let the pressure release naturally.

6. Open the Instant Pot and add the barley. Use the slow cooker function on the Instant Pot, affix the lid (vent open), and continue to cook for 1 hour until the barley is cooked through and tender. Serve.

❧

Option tip: **If you don't have either an Instant Pot or a slow cooker, you can also make this on the stove top. In a large pot, heat the oil over medium-high heat, sear the meat on all sides, remove it from the pan, and set aside. Add the mushrooms to the pan and cook briefly for 1 or 2 minutes. Remove and set aside. Add the onions, carrot, and celery to the pot and sauté until they are softened. Add the garlic and sauté until fragrant. Add the beef and mushrooms back to the pan, along with the thyme, beef broth, and water. Bring to a boil, reduce the heat, and simmer, covered, for 1½ to 2 hours until the meat just begins to get tender. Add the pearl barley and cook for an additional 30 to 40 minutes until it is tender. If needed, add up to 1 more cup water during cooking to achieve the desired consistency.**

Complete the Plate: **This hearty soup contains veggies, protein, and carbs, but you may find yourself needing more. I recommend serving with a sandwich or salad. Personally, I love the Red Pepper, Goat Cheese, and Arugula Open-Faced Grilled Sandwich (page 113), as it is a quick and easy addition to any meal.**

PER SERVING: Calories: 245; Total Fat: 9g; Protein: 21g; Carbohydrates: 19g; Sugars: 3g; Fiber: 4g; Sodium: 516mg

Cucumber, Tomato, and Avocado Salad

Gluten-Free | Vegan | Dairy-Free | Nut-Free | No-Cook | 30 Minutes or Less

The key to creating wonderful and nutritious food that you will come back to again and again is flavor. In this salad, dill brings a bright, unexpected touch to the otherwise ordinary combination of tomato, cucumber, and avocado. This salad pairs well with a protein-rich soup, such as Chicken Tortilla Soup (page 97), or Ceviche (page 199).

CARBS PER SERVING: 11g

SERVINGS: 4

PREP TIME: 10 minutes

1 cup cherry tomatoes, halved

1 large cucumber, chopped

1 small red onion, thinly sliced

1 avocado, diced

2 tablespoons chopped fresh dill

2 tablespoons extra-virgin olive oil

Juice of 1 lemon

¼ teaspoon salt

¼ teaspoon freshly ground black pepper

1. In a large mixing bowl, combine the tomatoes, cucumber, onion, avocado, and dill.

2. In a small bowl, combine the oil, lemon juice, salt, and pepper, and mix well.

3. Drizzle the dressing over the vegetables and toss to combine. Serve.

Substitution tip: If you don't have a lemon on hand, substitute 1 tablespoon red wine vinegar.

 Complete the Plate: This salad is perfect with Tuna, Hummus, and Veggie Wraps (page 115) or Black Bean Enchilada Skillet Casserole (page 135).

PER SERVING: Calories: 151; Total Fat: 12g; Protein: 2g; Carbohydrates: 11g; Sugars: 4g; Fiber: 4g; Sodium: 128mg

Cabbage Slaw Salad

Gluten-Free | Vegetarian | Dairy-Free | Nut-Free | No-Cook | 5-Ingredient
30 Minutes or Less

Even though I grew up in the South, I was never much of a coleslaw fan . . . until I realized I could make it myself. While commercial and restaurant versions usually have too much added sugar, I've found fresh, homemade versions to be healthier and a lot more flavorful. This one certainly won't disappoint.

CARBS PER SERVING: 10g
SERVINGS: 6
PREP TIME: 15 minutes

2 cups finely chopped green cabbage

2 cups finely chopped red cabbage

2 cups grated carrots

3 scallions, both white and green parts, sliced

2 tablespoons extra-virgin olive oil

2 tablespoons rice vinegar

1 teaspoon honey

1 garlic clove, minced

¼ teaspoon salt

1. In a large bowl, toss together the green and red cabbage, carrots, and scallions.

2. In a small bowl, whisk together the oil, vinegar, honey, garlic, and salt.

3. Pour the dressing over the veggies and mix to thoroughly combine.

4. Serve immediately, or cover and chill for several hours before serving.

Option tip: Add ¼ cup hemp seeds or ¼ cup pepitas to the slaw to increase the protein to 14g (hemp seeds) or 4g (pepitas).

Complete the Plate: This is the perfect dish to serve on top or alongside Barbecue Turkey Burger Sliders (page 170).

PER SERVING: Calories: 80; Total Fat: 5g; Protein: 1g; Carbohydrates: 10g; Sugars: 6g; Fiber: 3g; Sodium: 126mg

Green Salad with Blackberries, Goat Cheese, and Sweet Potatoes

Gluten-Free | Vegetarian | Nut-Free

Having a wide variety of salads to pull from for your everyday meal planning ensures that you won't get stuck in a salad rut. This fun salad combines blackberries with sweet and salty sweet potatoes and goat cheese for a well-balanced and taste-bud-loving combination. To save time on prep, make the vinaigrette and roast the sweet potato up to 1 day in advance, and assemble the remaining ingredients directly before serving.

CARBS PER SERVING: 21g

SERVINGS: 4

PREP TIME: 15 minutes

COOK TIME: 20 minutes

FOR THE VINAIGRETTE

1 pint blackberries

2 tablespoons red wine vinegar

1 tablespoon honey

3 tablespoons extra-virgin olive oil

¼ teaspoon salt

Freshly ground black pepper

FOR THE SALAD

1 sweet potato, cubed

1 teaspoon extra-virgin olive oil

8 cups salad greens (baby spinach, spicy greens, romaine)

½ red onion, sliced

¼ cup crumbled goat cheese

TO MAKE THE VINAIGRETTE

In a blender jar, combine the blackberries, vinegar, honey, oil, salt, and pepper, and process until smooth. Set aside.

TO MAKE THE SALAD

1. Preheat the oven to 425°F. Line a baking sheet with parchment paper.
2. In a medium mixing bowl, toss the sweet potato with the olive oil. Transfer to the prepared baking sheet and roast for 20 minutes, stirring once halfway through, until tender. Remove and cool for a few minutes.
3. In a large bowl, toss the greens with the red onion and cooled sweet potato, and drizzle with the vinaigrette. Serve topped with 1 tablespoon of goat cheese per serving.

Option tip: **For more protein, add 1 or 2 tablespoons hemp seeds to the dressing, along with a tablespoon or two of water to achieve the desired consistency.**

 Complete the Plate: **Serve alongside an easy protein like Roasted Salmon with Honey-Mustard Sauce (page 194) or Ginger-Garlic Cod Cooked in Paper (page 202).**

PER SERVING: Calories: 196; Total Fat: 12g; Protein: 3g; Carbohydrates: 21g; Sugars: 10g; Fiber: 6g; Sodium: 184mg

Three Bean and Basil Salad

Gluten-Free | Vegetarian | Dairy-Free | Nut-Free | No-Cook | 30 Minutes or Less

Beans are about 20 percent protein and are a good source of calcium, potassium, iron, zinc, and B vitamins. While they also contain carbohydrates, they have a whopping 7 to 8 grams of fiber per ½ cup, so the carbs are more slowly digested in the body, thus ensuring their impact on blood sugar levels are minimal. As long as you keep an eye on your serving size, you can enjoy this classic three-bean salad regularly.

CARBS PER SERVING: 29g
SERVINGS: 8
PREP TIME: 10 minutes

1 (15-ounce) can low-sodium chickpeas, drained and rinsed

1 (15-ounce) can low-sodium kidney beans, drained and rinsed

1 (15-ounce) can low-sodium white beans, drained and rinsed

1 red bell pepper, seeded and finely chopped

¼ cup chopped scallions, both white and green parts

¼ cup finely chopped fresh basil

3 garlic cloves, minced

2 tablespoons extra-virgin olive oil

1 tablespoon red wine vinegar

1 teaspoon Dijon mustard

¼ teaspoon freshly ground black pepper

1. In a large mixing bowl, combine the chickpeas, kidney beans, white beans, bell pepper, scallions, basil, and garlic. Toss gently to combine.

2. In a small bowl, combine the olive oil, vinegar, mustard, and pepper. Toss with the salad.

3. Cover and refrigerate for an hour before serving, to allow the flavors to mix.

Substitution tip: **Feel free to substitute home-cooked beans in place of canned, using about 1½ cups per variety.**

Complete the Plate: **This isn't a stand-alone meal, so definitely add another serving of vegetables, healthy fat, and a 2- to 3-ounce portion of protein. A great choice is Tuna, Hummus, and Veggie Wraps (page 115) or Herbed Chicken Meatball Wraps (page 117).**

PER SERVING: Calories: 193; Total Fat: 5g; Protein: 10g; Carbohydrates: 29g; Sugars: 3g; Fiber: 8g; Sodium: 246mg

Rainbow Black Bean Salad

Gluten-Free | Vegetarian | Dairy-Free | Nut-Free | No-Cook | 30 Minutes or Less

This Mexican-style salad is beautiful to the eye, with bright red bell peppers and cherry tomatoes, vibrant green spinach, scallions, crunchy jicama, and avocado. It's topped with a lime-and-garlic vinaigrette whose bright flavor wonderfully ties it all together.

CARBS PER SERVING: 22g

SERVINGS: 5

PREP TIME: 15 minutes

1 (15-ounce) can low-sodium black beans, drained and rinsed

1 avocado, diced

1 cup cherry tomatoes, halved

1 cup chopped baby spinach

½ cup finely chopped red bell pepper

¼ cup finely chopped jicama

½ cup chopped scallions, both white and green parts

¼ cup chopped fresh cilantro

2 tablespoons freshly squeezed lime juice

1 tablespoon extra-virgin olive oil

2 garlic cloves, minced

1 teaspoon honey

¼ teaspoon salt

¼ teaspoon freshly ground black pepper

1. In a large bowl, combine the black beans, avocado, tomatoes, spinach, bell pepper, jicama, scallions, and cilantro.

2. In a small bowl, mix the lime juice, oil, garlic, honey, salt, and pepper. Add to the salad and toss.

3. Chill for 1 hour before serving.

Option tip: For a little kick of heat in the salad, add a minced jalapeño or serrano pepper to the vinaigrette.

 Complete the Plate: Serve this salad on the side of a bowl of Chicken Tortilla Soup (page 97) or with your favorite protein such as Roasted Salmon with Salsa Verde (page 197) or Tomato Tuna Melts (page 192).

PER SERVING: Calories: 169; Total Fat: 7g; Protein: 6g; Carbohydrates: 22g; Sugars: 3g; Fiber: 9g; Sodium: 235mg

Warm Barley and Squash Salad with Balsamic Vinaigrette

Vegan | Dairy-Free

Butternut squash is easy to prepare and has a naturally sweet, creamy taste that works well in so many dishes. Packed with vitamins A and C, squash even has anticancer properties that make it a valuable addition to your meals.

CARBS PER SERVING: 32g

SERVINGS: 8

PREP TIME: 20 minutes

COOK TIME: 40 minutes

1 small butternut squash

3 teaspoons plus
2 tablespoons extra-virgin olive oil, divided

2 cups broccoli florets

1 cup pearl barley

1 cup toasted
chopped walnuts

2 cups baby kale

½ red onion, sliced

2 tablespoons
balsamic vinegar

2 garlic cloves, minced

½ teaspoon salt

¼ teaspoon freshly ground black pepper

1. Preheat the oven to 400°F. Line a baking sheet with parchment paper.

2. Peel and seed the squash, and cut it into dice. In a large bowl, toss the squash with 2 teaspoons of olive oil. Transfer to the prepared baking sheet and roast for 20 minutes.

3. While the squash is roasting, toss the broccoli in the same bowl with 1 teaspoon of olive oil. After 20 minutes, flip the squash and push it to one side of the baking sheet. Add the broccoli to the other side and continue to roast for 20 more minutes until tender.

4. While the veggies are roasting, in a medium pot, cover the barley with several inches of water. Bring to a boil, then reduce the heat, cover, and simmer for 30 minutes until tender. Drain and rinse.

5. Transfer the barley to a large bowl, and toss with the cooked squash and broccoli, walnuts, kale, and onion.

6. In a small bowl, mix the remaining 2 tablespoons of olive oil, balsamic vinegar, garlic, salt, and pepper. Toss the salad with the dressing and serve.

◆➤

Ingredient tip: Butternut squash is one of the simplest winter squashes to prepare because its tough outer layer is easy to remove. Cut off one end of the squash so it stands upright on the cut end. Using a sharp knife or a vegetable peeler, start at the top of the squash and cut the skin off downward in strips, working around the squash, until it's peeled.

Complete the Plate: Add another protein source to complete this plate. You can simply grill or bake 2 or 3 ounces of your favorite lean protein at the same time you are roasting the butternut squash.

PER SERVING: Calories: 274; Total Fat: 15g; Protein: 6g; Carbohydrates: 32g; Sugars: 3g; Fiber: 7g; Sodium: 144mg

Winter Chicken and Citrus Salad

Gluten-Free | Dairy-Free | No-Cook | 30 Minutes or Less

Citrus may seem like an unlikely salad ingredient, but they're at the peak of freshness during the winter and are loaded with vitamin C, which helps naturally improve your immune system if a winter cold strikes. Finished with a lemon vinaigrette, this salad is perfectly refreshing.

CARBS PER SERVING: 11g

SERVINGS: 4

PREP TIME: 10 minutes

4 cups baby spinach

2 tablespoons extra-virgin olive oil

1 tablespoon freshly squeezed lemon juice

⅛ teaspoon salt

Freshly ground black pepper

2 cups chopped cooked chicken

2 mandarin oranges, peeled and sectioned

½ peeled grapefruit, sectioned

¼ cup sliced almonds

1. In a large mixing bowl, toss the spinach with the olive oil, lemon juice, salt, and pepper.

2. Add the chicken, oranges, grapefruit, and almonds to the bowl. Toss gently.

3. Arrange on 4 plates and serve.

Ingredient tip: While grapefruit contains powerful and helpful nutrients, it also contains a naturally occurring chemical that interferes with your body's ability to break down cholesterol-lowering statin medications. If you are taking any of these medications, be sure to skip the grapefruit in this recipe.

Complete the Plate: **Complete the plate by serving with Comforting Summer Squash Soup with Crispy Chickpeas (page 92) or Curried Carrot Soup (page 94).**

PER SERVING: Calories: 249; Total Fat: 12g; Protein: 24g; Carbohydrates: 11g; Sugars: 7g; Fiber: 3g; Sodium: 135mg

Blueberry and Chicken Salad
on a Bed of Greens

Gluten-Free | No-Cook | 30 Minutes or Less

Chicken salad is a great lunch, especially when its nutritional value is increased by adding antioxidant-rich fresh blueberries to the mix. Trade in the bread for a bed of salad greens, and you have an easy and filling lunch that anyone will enjoy.

CARBS PER SERVING: 11g

SERVINGS: 4

PREP TIME: 10 minutes

2 cups chopped
cooked chicken

1 cup fresh blueberries

¼ cup finely
chopped almonds

1 celery stalk, finely chopped

¼ cup finely chopped
red onion

1 tablespoon chopped
fresh basil

1 tablespoon chopped fresh
cilantro

½ cup plain, nonfat Greek
yogurt or vegan mayonnaise

¼ teaspoon salt

¼ teaspoon freshly ground
black pepper

8 cups salad greens (baby
spinach, spicy greens,
romaine)

1. In a large mixing bowl, combine the chicken, blueberries, almonds, celery, onion, basil, and cilantro. Toss gently to mix.

2. In a small bowl, combine the yogurt, salt, and pepper. Add to the chicken salad and stir to combine.

3. Arrange 2 cups of salad greens on each of 4 plates and divide the chicken salad among the plates to serve.

Make-ahead tip: **Make the chicken salad up to 3 days in advance and store refrigerated in an airtight container until ready to serve with the greens.**

Complete the Plate: I love topping this salad with a few slices of avocado to add some satisfying healthy fats, and adding a serving of whole-wheat crackers (my favorite brands are Ak-Mak and Wasa).

PER SERVING: Calories: 207; Total Fat: 6g; Protein: 28g; Carbohydrates: 11g; Sugars: 6g; Fiber: 3g; Sodium: 235mg

Salmon, Quinoa, and Avocado Salad

Gluten-Free | Dairy-Free | Nut-Free

Quinoa is often thought of as a grain, but it is actually a seed. It's frequently referred to as a superfood because it contains fiber-rich carbs, protein, and many health-promoting vitamins and nutrients, making it a great substitute for rice. Quinoa is also a fabulous source of magnesium, which is commonly low in people with diabetes, so it's especially helpful for anyone who is newly diagnosed.

CARBS PER SERVING: 23g

SERVINGS: 4

PREP TIME: 15 minutes

COOK TIME: 20 minutes

½ cup quinoa

1 cup water

4 (4-ounce) salmon fillets

1 pound asparagus, trimmed

1 teaspoon extra-virgin olive oil, plus 2 tablespoons

½ teaspoon salt, divided

½ teaspoon freshly ground black pepper, divided

¼ teaspoon red pepper flakes

1 avocado, chopped

¼ cup chopped scallions, both white and green parts

¼ cup chopped fresh cilantro

1 tablespoon minced fresh oregano

Juice of 1 lime

1. In a small pot, combine the quinoa and water, and bring to a boil over medium-high heat. Cover, reduce the heat, and simmer for 15 minutes.

2. Preheat the oven to 425°F. Line a large baking sheet with parchment paper.

3. Arrange the salmon on one side of the prepared baking sheet. Toss the asparagus with 1 teaspoon of olive oil, and arrange on the other side of the baking sheet. Season the salmon and asparagus with ¼ teaspoon of salt, ¼ teaspoon of pepper, and the red pepper flakes. Roast for 12 minutes until browned and cooked through.

4. While the fish and asparagus are cooking, in a large mixing bowl, gently toss the cooked quinoa, avocado, scallions, cilantro, and oregano. Add the remaining 2 tablespoons of olive oil and the lime juice, and season with the remaining ¼ teaspoon of salt and ¼ teaspoon of pepper.

◆→

5. Break the salmon into pieces, removing the skin and any bones, and chop the asparagus into bite-sized pieces. Fold into the quinoa and serve warm or at room temperature.

Make-ahead tip: Make the quinoa, roast the salmon, and prepare the scallions, cilantro, and oregano the night before to make it easy to throw this salad together for a quick lunch before leaving the house in the morning.

PER SERVING: Calories: 397; Total Fat: 22g; Protein: 29g; Carbohydrates: 23g; Sugars: 3g; Fiber: 8g; Sodium: 292mg

Red Pepper, Goat Cheese, and Arugula Open-Faced Grilled Sandwich

Vegetarian | Nut-Free | 5-Ingredient | 30 Minutes or Less

Upgrade your traditional grilled cheese sandwich with this veggie-filled open-faced version. Bell peppers are my absolute favorite vegetable, so I am always adding them to anything and everything I'm eating. You will be pleasantly surprised by how easy this sandwich is to make, while adding a gourmet touch to your meals.

CARBS PER SERVING: 21g
SERVINGS: 1
PREP TIME: 5 minutes
COOK TIME: 15 minutes

½ red bell pepper, seeded

Nonstick cooking spray

1 slice whole-wheat thin-sliced bread (I love Ezekiel sprouted bread and Dave's Killer Bread)

2 tablespoons crumbled goat cheese

Pinch dried thyme

½ cup arugula

1. Preheat the broiler to high. Line a baking sheet with parchment paper.

2. Cut the ½ bell pepper lengthwise into two pieces and arrange on the prepared baking sheet with the skin facing up.

3. Broil for 5 to 10 minutes until the skin is blackened. Transfer to a covered container to steam for 5 minutes, then remove the skin from the pepper using your fingers. Cut the pepper into strips.

4. Heat a small skillet over medium-high heat. Spray it with nonstick cooking spray and place the bread in the skillet. Top with the goat cheese and sprinkle with the thyme. Pile the arugula on top, followed by the roasted red pepper strips. Press down with a spatula to hold in place.

➤

5. Cook for 2 to 3 minutes until the bread is crisp and browned and the cheese is warmed through. (If you prefer, you can make a half-closed sandwich instead: Cut the bread in half and place one half in the skillet. Top with the cheese, thyme, arugula, red pepper, and the other half slice of bread. Cook for 4 to 6 minutes, flipping once, until both sides are browned.)

Substitution tip: **Substitute any tender mild greens, such as spinach or a baby green salad mix, for the arugula.**

 Complete the Plate: **Serve with a soup or salad, like Chicken Tortilla Soup (page 97) or Winter Chicken and Citrus Salad (page 109).**

PER SERVING: Calories: 109; Total Fat: 2g; Protein: 4g; Carbohydrates: 21g; Sugars: 5g; Fiber: 6g; Sodium: 123mg

Tuna, Hummus, and Veggie Wraps

Gluten-Free | Dairy-Free | Nut-Free | No-Cook | 30 Minutes or Less

Making homemade hummus is so much easier than you might think, and it will ensure you aren't eating the unwanted additives many commercial varieties contain. You can use low-sodium canned chickpeas here, or cook your own. One wrap makes a great energy-boosting snack for any time of the day, or have two for a main meal. Whatever works best for you!

CARBS PER SERVING: 15g
SERVINGS: 2 (2 wraps each), plus extra hummus
PREP TIME: 10 minutes

FOR THE HUMMUS

1 cup from 1 (15-ounce) can low-sodium chickpeas, drained and rinsed

2 tablespoons tahini

1 tablespoon extra-virgin olive oil

1 garlic clove

Juice of ½ lemon

¼ teaspoon salt

2 tablespoons water

FOR THE WRAPS

4 large lettuce leaves

1 (5-ounce) can chunk light tuna packed in water, drained

1 red bell pepper, seeded and cut into strips

1 cucumber, sliced

TO MAKE THE HUMMUS

In a blender jar, combine the chickpeas, tahini, olive oil, garlic, lemon juice, salt, and water. Process until smooth. Taste and adjust with additional lemon juice or salt, as needed.

TO MAKE THE WRAPS

1. On each lettuce leaf, spread 1 tablespoon of hummus, and divide the tuna among the leaves. Top each with several strips of red pepper and cucumber slices.

2. Roll up the lettuce leaves, folding in the two shorter sides and rolling away from you, like a burrito. Serve.

Make-ahead tip: **Make the hummus up to 3 days in advance and store in a covered container in the refrigerator.**

Complete the Plate: **While this recipe meets the balanced-plate requirements, consider adding an extra veggie serving and another carb choice, such as a whole piece of fruit.**

PER SERVING: Calories: 191; Total Fat: 5g; Protein: 26g; Carbohydrates: 15g; Sugars: 6g; Fiber: 4g; Sodium: 357mg

Thai-Style Chicken Roll-Ups

Dairy-Free | No-Cook | 30 Minutes or Less

I look forward to the Thai-inspired flavors of this recipe every week. This is one of my personal favorite go-to lunches. I highly recommend prepping the ingredients on the weekend, so you can throw this together in less than 5 minutes before work during your busy week.

CARBS PER SERVING: 17g

SERVINGS: 4

PREP TIME: 15 minutes

1½ cups shredded cooked chicken breast

1 cup bean sprouts

1 cup shredded green cabbage

½ cup shredded carrots

¼ cup chopped scallions, both white and green parts

¼ cup chopped fresh cilantro

2 tablespoons natural peanut butter

2 tablespoons water

1 tablespoon rice wine vinegar

1 garlic clove, minced

¼ teaspoon salt

4 (8-inch) low-carb whole-wheat tortillas

1. In a large mixing bowl, toss the chicken breast, bean sprouts, cabbage, carrots, scallions, and cilantro.

2. In a medium bowl, whisk together the peanut butter, water, rice vinegar, garlic, and salt.

3. Fill each tortilla with about 1 cup of the chicken and vegetable mixture, and spoon a tablespoon of sauce over the filling.

4. Fold in two opposite sides of the tortilla and roll up. Serve.

Substitution tip: For a lighter wrap, use large lettuce leaves in place of the tortillas, or simply serve the dish as a salad.

 Complete the Plate: This is a balanced meal, but I would recommend adding another serving of vegetables and another serving of carbohydrates, such as your favorite fruit.

PER SERVING: Calories: 210; Total Fat: 8g; Protein: 21g; Carbohydrates: 17g; Sugars: 3g; Fiber: 10g; Sodium: 360mg

Herbed Chicken Meatball Wraps

Gluten-Free | Nut-Free | 30 Minutes or Less

Enjoy these fresh, Mediterranean-inspired meatballs paired with crispy lettuce leaves for a nutrient-dense and flavorful meal. Not only are these meatballs easy to make, they can be frozen to provide a backup meal for the days when you are running short on time.

CARBS PER SERVING: 6g

SERVINGS: 6

(2 wraps each)

PREP TIME: 10 minutes

COOK TIME: 20 minutes

1 pound ground chicken

3 scallions, both white and green parts, finely chopped

2 garlic cloves, minced

2 tablespoons chopped fresh mint

½ teaspoon dried oregano

1 egg, lightly beaten

12 large lettuce leaves

1 medium red bell pepper, seeded and cut into strips

1 carrot, cut into strips

1 recipe Cucumber-Yogurt Dip (page 235)

1. Preheat the oven to 400°F. Line a baking sheet with parchment paper.

2. In a large mixing bowl, combine the chicken, scallions, garlic, mint, oregano, and egg. Stir well.

3. Using your hands, form the meat mixture into balls about the size of a tablespoon, making about 24 balls. Arrange on the prepared baking sheet.

4. Bake for 10 minutes, flip with a spatula, and continue baking for an additional 10 minutes until the meatballs are cooked through.

5. In each lettuce leaf, place two meatballs and several bell pepper and carrot strips. Top with 2 tablespoons of Cucumber-Yogurt Dip. Wrap the leaves around the filling and serve with the dip.

Substitution tip: You can use ground turkey instead of chicken. And if you don't like lettuce wraps, feel free to substitute whole-wheat tortillas or wraps.

Complete the Plate: Add another serving of carbohydrates and veggies to make this a more complete plate. My favorite addition is Cucumber, Tomato, and Avocado Salad (page 101).

PER SERVING: Calories: 220; Total Fat: 12g; Protein: 23g; Carbohydrates: 6g; Sugars: 3g; Fiber: 2g; Sodium: 199mg

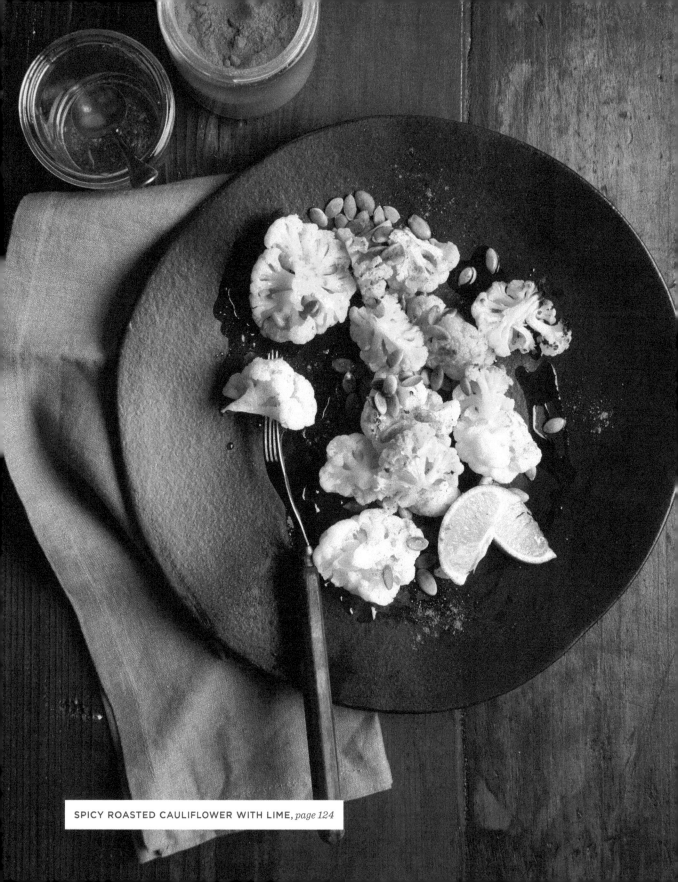

SPICY ROASTED CAULIFLOWER WITH LIME, *page 124*

8

Vegetable Side Dishes

Sautéed Spinach and Tomatoes

Gluten-Free | Vegan | Dairy-Free | Nut-Free | 5-Ingredient | 30 Minutes or Less

Spinach is one of the most widely available greens and also one of the most nutritionally packed. Loaded with iron, calcium, lutein, vitamin K, folic acid, and carotenes, the mild-flavored powerhouse is easy to incorporate into your diet regularly. In this easy dish, it is mixed with sweet cherry tomatoes for simple yet surprisingly delicious results.

CARBS PER SERVING: 4g
SERVINGS: 4
PREP TIME: 5 minutes
COOK TIME: 10 minutes

1 tablespoon extra-virgin olive oil

1 cup cherry tomatoes, halved

3 spinach bunches, trimmed

2 garlic cloves, minced

¼ teaspoon salt

1. In a large skillet, heat the oil over medium heat.

2. Add the tomatoes, and cook until the skins begin to blister and split, about 2 minutes.

3. Add the spinach in batches, waiting for each batch to wilt slightly before adding the next batch. Stir continuously for 3 to 4 minutes until the spinach is tender.

4. Add the garlic to the skillet, and toss until fragrant, about 30 seconds.

5. Drain the excess liquid from the pan. Add the salt. Stir well and serve.

Option tip: Add a pinch or two of red pepper flakes to turn up the heat of this recipe.

PER SERVING: Calories: 52; Total Fat: 4g; Protein: 2g; Carbohydrates: 4g; Sugars: 1g; Fiber: 2g; Sodium: 183mg

Garlicky Cabbage and Collard Greens

Gluten-Free | Vegan | Dairy-Free | Nut-Free | 5-Ingredient | 30 Minutes or Less

Leafy greens are a nutrient-dense addition to any meal and are something that should be on your table several times a week. This simple preparation is quick and flavorful. Loaded with calcium and vitamin C, collards are nature's own medicine cabinet, with anticancer, antiviral, antibiotic, and antioxidant properties. Cabbage, also a nutritional powerhouse loaded with vitamin C, is sweeter and a perfect pairing with the collards.

CARBS PER SERVING: 6g

SERVINGS: 8

PREP TIME: 10 minutes

COOK TIME: 10 minutes

2 tablespoons extra-virgin olive oil

1 collard greens bunch, stemmed and thinly sliced

½ small green cabbage, thinly sliced

6 garlic cloves, minced

1 tablespoon low-sodium gluten-free soy sauce or tamari

1. In a large skillet, heat the oil over medium-high heat.

2. Add the collards to the pan, stirring to coat with oil. Sauté for 1 to 2 minutes until the greens begin to wilt.

3. Add the cabbage and stir to coat. Cover and reduce the heat to medium low. Continue to cook for 5 to 7 minutes, stirring once or twice, until the greens are tender.

4. Add the garlic and soy sauce and stir to incorporate. Cook until just fragrant, about 30 seconds longer. Serve warm and enjoy!

Technique tip: When cooking collards this way, it is important to remove the tough stems to enable quick cooking. To quickly prep collards without a knife, place each collard green on a work surface and fold it over so that the stem is facing you. Holding the leafy part in place with one hand, use your other hand to pull the stem upward and away from the green.

PER SERVING: Calories: 72; Total Fat: 4g; Protein: 3g; Carbohydrates: 6g; Sugars: 0g; Fiber: 3g; Sodium: 129mg

Roasted Lemon and Garlic Broccoli

Gluten-Free | Vegan | Dairy-Free | Nut-Free | 5-Ingredient

Roasting broccoli is one of the best ways to enhance its natural flavor. Garlic and lemon juice make this simple side a favorite and something you can keep coming back to again and again. Pair it with fish, chicken, or vegetable dishes for a filling and vitamin C–rich side.

CARBS PER SERVING: 3g
SERVINGS: 8
PREP TIME: 10 minutes
COOK TIME: 25 minutes

2 large broccoli heads, cut into florets

3 garlic cloves, minced

2 tablespoons extra-virgin olive oil

¼ teaspoon salt

¼ teaspoon freshly ground black pepper

2 tablespoons freshly squeezed lemon juice

1. Preheat the oven to 425°F.

2. On a rimmed baking sheet, toss the broccoli, garlic, and olive oil. Season with the salt and pepper.

3. Roast, tossing occasionally, for 25 to 30 minutes until tender and browned. Season with the lemon juice and serve.

Substitution tip: This same preparation works well with Brussels sprouts, cauliflower, and even broccoli rabe.

PER SERVING: Calories: 30; Total Fat: 2g; Protein: 1g; Carbohydrates: 3g; Sugars: 1g; Fiber: 1g; Sodium: 84mg

Cauli-Broccoli Tots

Vegetarian | Nut-Free | 30 Minutes or Less

Tater tots were a childhood favorite for many of us growing up. But since I've become a mom, I know adding more veggies is important for adults and kids alike. Because you are processing the broccoli and cauliflower in a food processor stems can be used too, making this a perfect way to cut food waste and use up any extra stems you have after cutting florets from heads. Serve these straight out of the oven for the best flavor.

CARBS PER SERVING: 9g
SERVINGS: 4
PREP TIME: 10 minutes
COOK TIME: 20 minutes

1 cup chopped broccoli florets and stems

1 cup chopped cauliflower florets and stems

¼ cup diced onion

1 large egg

¼ cup whole-wheat bread crumbs

¼ cup crumbled feta cheese

½ teaspoon salt

¼ teaspoon freshly ground black pepper

1. Preheat the oven to 400°F. Line a baking sheet with parchment paper.

2. In a food processor, combine the broccoli, cauliflower, and onion, and pulse until chopped well but still slightly chunky. Or if you don't have a food processor, chop everything on a large cutting board until you have very small pieces. Transfer to a large mixing bowl.

3. Add the egg, bread crumbs, cheese, salt, and pepper.

4. Using your hands, shape small balls, a little smaller than a tablespoon, and carefully place them on the prepared baking sheet.

5. Bake for 10 minutes, flip carefully, and continue to bake for 10 additional minutes until browned and crisp.

Technique tip: Save time on shaping the tots by spraying a mini muffin tin with nonstick cooking spray and lightly pressing the mixture into the cups, then baking as directed.

PER SERVING: Calories: 90; Total Fat: 4g; Protein: 5g; Carbohydrates: 9g; Sugars: 2g; Fiber: 2g; Sodium: 424mg

Spicy Roasted Cauliflower with Lime

Gluten-Free | Vegan | Dairy-Free | Nut-Free | 5-Ingredient | 30 Minutes or Less

I haven't always been a cauliflower lover. But as I've discovered its versatility—it's able to take on the flavor of whatever it is paired with while being a simple, lower-carb substitution—it's now become one of the veggies I recommend the most. Like so many other vegetables, roasting brings out the sweetness of the cauliflower and transforms it into a crave-worthy side dish.

CARBS PER SERVING: 8g
SERVINGS: 4
PREP TIME: 5 minutes
COOK TIME: 10 minutes

1 cauliflower head, broken into small florets

2 tablespoons extra-virgin olive oil

½ teaspoon ground chipotle chili powder

½ teaspoon salt

Juice of 1 lime

1. Preheat the oven to 450°F. Line a rimmed baking sheet with parchment paper.

2. In a large mixing bowl, toss the cauliflower with the olive oil, chipotle chili powder, and salt. Arrange in a single layer on the prepared baking sheet.

3. Roast for 15 minutes, flip, and continue to roast for 15 more minutes until well-browned and tender.

4. Sprinkle with the lime juice, adjust the salt as needed, and serve.

Ingredient tip: Chipotle chili powder is a mild chili powder that lends a smoky flavor to foods. Find it at specialty spice shops and well-stocked grocery stores.

PER SERVING: Calories: 99; Total Fat: 7g; Protein: 3g; Carbohydrates: 8g; Sugars: 3g; Fiber: 3g; Sodium: 284mg

Roasted Delicata Squash

Gluten-Free | Vegan | Dairy-Free | Nut-Free | 5-Ingredient | 30 Minutes or Less

Delicata squash, a winter squash that resembles a plump yellow cucumber, is lightly sweet and quite creamy when cooked. Because it has thin skin, the squash does not require peeling, making it a perfect side dish on a busy night. This simple roasted preparation pairs well with meat and vegetarian dishes alike. Because delicata squash is a winter squash, it is higher in carbs than summer squash, so feel free to swap for a less starchy squash if you desire.

CARBS PER SERVING: 12g
SERVINGS: 4
PREP TIME: 10 minutes
COOK TIME: 20 minutes

1 (1- to 1½-pound) delicata squash, halved, seeded, cut into ½-inch-thick strips

1 tablespoon extra-virgin olive oil

½ teaspoon dried thyme

¼ teaspoon salt

¼ teaspoon freshly ground black pepper

1. Preheat the oven to 400°F. Line a baking sheet with parchment paper.

2. In a large mixing bowl, toss the squash strips with the olive oil, thyme, salt, and pepper. Arrange on the prepared baking sheet in a single layer.

3. Roast for 10 minutes, flip, and continue to roast for 10 more minutes until tender and lightly browned.

Substitution tip: Use rosemary, cinnamon, or oregano in place of the thyme for a different flavor.

PER SERVING: Calories: 79; Total Fat: 4g; Protein: 1g; Carbohydrates: 12g; Sugars: 3g; Fiber: 2g; Sodium: 123mg

Roasted Asparagus, Onions, and Red Peppers

Gluten-Free | Vegetarian | Dairy-Free | Nut-Free | 5-Ingredient | 30 Minutes or Less

The great thing about roasting vegetables is that you can set them in the oven and go about preparing the other parts of the meal while they cook. This recipe is the perfect addition to any Italian dish. Look for uniformly sized bunches of asparagus when purchasing, for even cooking.

CARBS PER SERVING: 11g

SERVINGS: 4

PREP TIME: 5 minutes

COOK TIME: 20 minutes

1 pound asparagus, woody ends trimmed, cut into 2-inch segments

1 small onion, quartered

2 red bell peppers, seeded, cut into 1-inch pieces

2 tablespoons Easy Italian Dressing (page 238)

1. Preheat the oven to 400°F. Line a baking sheet with parchment paper.

2. In a large mixing bowl, toss the asparagus, onion, and peppers with the dressing. Transfer to the prepared baking sheet.

3. Roast for 10 minutes, then, using a spatula, flip the vegetables. Roast for 5 to 10 more minutes until the vegetables are tender.

4. Stir well and serve.

Option tip: **For a little spice, add slices of jalapeño peppers to the mixture in step 2.**

PER SERVING: Calories: 93; Total Fat: 5g; Protein: 3g; Carbohydrates: 11g; Sugars: 6g; Fiber: 4g; Sodium: 32mg

Green Bean Casserole

Vegan | Dairy-Free

When I was growing up in Tennessee, there were few family gatherings that didn't include this classic Southern staple. Over time, I realized that it was so easy to make my own "cream of mushroom" addition to this casserole to give it even more flavor and provide additional nutrients, without the unwanted sodium. You can find almond flour with the other flours in some grocery stores or with the fancy grain products. Or look for it in a health food store. Enjoy this casserole around the table with those you love, knowing it is a healthy addition to any occasion.

CARBS PER SERVING: 7g
SERVINGS: 8
PREP TIME: 10 minutes
COOK TIME: 30 minutes

1 pound green beans, trimmed, cut into bite-size pieces

3 tablespoons extra-virgin olive oil, divided

8 ounces brown mushrooms, diced

3 garlic cloves, minced

1½ tablespoons whole-wheat flour

1 cup low-sodium vegetable broth

1 cup unsweetened plain almond milk

¼ cup almond flour

2 tablespoons dried minced onion

1. Preheat the oven to 400°F.

2. Bring a large pot of water to a boil. Boil the green beans for 3 to 5 minutes until just barely tender but still bright green. Drain and set aside.

3. In a medium skillet, heat 2 tablespoons of oil over medium-high heat. Add the mushrooms and stir. Cook for 3 to 5 minutes until the mushrooms brown and release their liquid. Add the garlic and stir until just fragrant, about 30 seconds.

4. Add the whole-wheat flour and stir well to combine. Add the broth and simmer for 1 minute.

5. Reduce the heat to medium low and add the almond milk. Return to a simmer and cook for 5 to 7 minutes until the mixture thickens.

➡

6. Remove from the heat. Stir in the green beans and transfer to a baking dish.

7. In a small bowl, mix the almond flour, dried minced onion, and remaining 1 tablespoon of olive oil, and stir until combined and crumbly. Crumble over the beans.

8. Bake for 15 to 20 minutes until the liquids are bubbling and the top is browned.

Make-ahead tip: Make the casserole 1 or 2 days ahead through step 6, and refrigerate, covered. When you are ready to cook, add the topping and increase the cooking time by about 10 minutes.

PER SERVING: Calories: 97; Total Fat: 7g; Protein: 2g; Carbohydrates: 7g; Sugars: 2g; Fiber: 2g; Sodium: 57mg

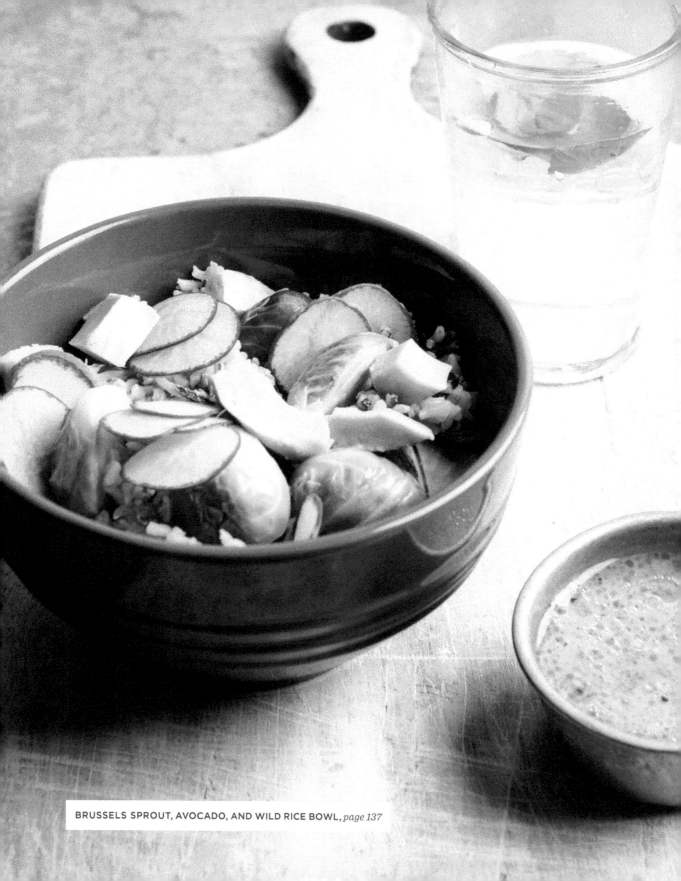

BRUSSELS SPROUT, AVOCADO, AND WILD RICE BOWL, *page 137*

9

Meatless Main Dishes

Beet, Goat Cheese, and Walnut Pesto with Zoodles

Gluten-Free | Vegetarian | 5-Ingredient

You're going to have to trust me on this recipe, because I'm sure it is like nothing you have ever tried before. The flavor is out of this world . . . and so are the colors! You might not be used to eating pink food, but I promise it is good for your health. Beets are rich in folate, fiber, and potassium. If you aren't a zoodle (zucchini noodle) lover yet, you can skip them and simply use the pesto as a dip for veggies or on top of your favorite simple green salad.

CARBS PER SERVING: 17g
SERVINGS: 2
PREP TIME: 15 minutes
COOK TIME: 40 minutes

1 medium red beet, peeled, chopped

½ cup walnut pieces

3 garlic cloves

½ cup crumbled goat cheese

2 tablespoons extra-virgin olive oil, plus 2 teaspoons

2 tablespoons freshly squeezed lemon juice

¼ teaspoon salt

4 small zucchini

1. Preheat the oven to 375°F.

2. Wrap the chopped beet in a piece of aluminum foil and seal well. Roast for 30 to 40 minutes until fork-tender.

3. Meanwhile, heat a dry skillet over medium-high heat. Toast the walnuts for 5 to 7 minutes until lightly browned and fragrant.

4. Transfer the cooked beets to the bowl of a food processor. Add the toasted walnuts, garlic, goat cheese, 2 tablespoons of olive oil, lemon juice, and salt. Process until smooth.

5. Using a spiralizer or sharp knife, cut the zucchini into thin "noodles."

6. In a large skillet, heat the remaining 2 teaspoons of oil over medium heat. Add the zucchini and toss in the oil. Cook, stirring gently, for 2 to 3 minutes, until the zucchini softens. Toss with the beet pesto and serve warm.

Substitution tip: If you don't like the distinctive taste of goat cheese, substitute grated Parmesan or crumbled feta cheese instead.

 Complete the Plate: This is a complete plate, but feel free to add a serving of your favorite lean protein, if you like.

PER SERVING: Calories: 422; Total Fat: 39g; Protein: 8g; Carbohydrates: 17g; Sugars: 10g; Fiber: 6g; Sodium: 339mg

Mushroom and Pesto Flatbread Pizza

Vegetarian | 5-Ingredient | 30 Minutes or Less

Pizza (thankfully!) doesn't have to be off-limits when it comes to eating with diabetes. Selecting quality ingredients goes a long way in creating a menu that you enjoy and that is right for you. Make these easy pizzas at home in minutes using a low-carb whole-wheat flatbread and store-bought pesto sauce. Just look for one with the least amount of sodium possible. Other vegetables, such as red and green bell peppers, spinach, artichoke hearts, sliced tomatoes, and olives, are all great toppings to add to this simple pizza. Pick your favorites and add them on. You will never feel deprived again!

CARBS PER SERVING: 28g

SERVINGS: 2

PREP TIME: 5 minutes

COOK TIME: 15 minutes

1 teaspoon extra-virgin olive oil

½ cup sliced mushrooms

½ red onion, sliced

Salt

Freshly ground black pepper

¼ cup store-bought pesto sauce

2 whole-wheat flatbreads

¼ cup shredded mozzarella cheese

1. Preheat the oven to 350°F.

2. In a small skillet, heat the oil over medium heat. Add the mushrooms and onion, and season with salt and pepper. Sauté for 3 to 5 minutes until the onion and mushrooms begin to soften.

3. Spread 2 tablespoons of pesto on each flatbread.

4. Divide the mushroom-onion mixture between the two flatbreads. Top each with 2 tablespoons of cheese.

5. Place the flatbreads on a baking sheet, and bake for 10 to 12 minutes until the cheese is melted and bubbly. Serve warm.

Ingredient tip: Flatbread is an unleavened bread similar to a pita but without a pocket. If you can't find flatbread, substitute an Ezekiel tortilla or a whole-wheat sandwich thin instead.

Complete the Plate: Enjoy an additional serving of veggies with this meal. I love starting with a simple salad topped with Easy Italian Dressing (page 238) or Miso-Ginger Dressing (page 237).

PER SERVING: Calories: 347; Total Fat: 23g; Protein: 14g; Carbohydrates: 28g; Sugars: 4g; Fiber: 7g; Sodium: 791mg

Black Bean Enchilada Skillet Casserole

Gluten-Free | Vegetarian | Nut-Free | 30 Minutes or Less

There is nothing better for a weeknight meal than a one-dish skillet casserole. Simple to throw together, this dish is loaded with flavor and packed with plenty of vegetable goodness. The best part? It's ready in half an hour, so it's the perfect go-to after a long day.

CARBS PER SERVING: 21g

SERVINGS: 6

PREP TIME: 15 minutes

COOK TIME: 15 minutes

1 tablespoon extra-virgin olive oil

½ onion, chopped

½ red bell pepper, seeded and chopped

½ green bell pepper, seeded and chopped

2 small zucchini, chopped

3 garlic cloves, minced

1 (15-ounce) can low-sodium black beans, drained and rinsed

1 (10-ounce) can low-sodium enchilada sauce

1 teaspoon ground cumin

¼ teaspoon salt

¼ teaspoon freshly ground black pepper

½ cup shredded cheddar cheese, divided

2 (6-inch) corn tortillas, cut into strips

Chopped fresh cilantro, for garnish

Plain yogurt, for serving

1. Heat the broiler to high.

2. In a large oven-safe skillet, heat the oil over medium-high heat.

3. Add the onion, red bell pepper, green bell pepper, zucchini, and garlic to the skillet, and cook for 3 to 5 minutes until the onion softens.

4. Add the black beans, enchilada sauce, cumin, salt, pepper, ¼ cup of cheese, and tortilla strips, and mix together. Top with the remaining ¼ cup of cheese.

5. Put the skillet under the broiler and broil for 5 to 8 minutes until the cheese is melted and bubbly. Garnish with cilantro and serve with yogurt on the side.

Option tip: To add some heat to the dish, add a minced jalapeño or serrano chile in step 3.

Complete the Plate: Add an extra protein such as Spice-Rubbed Crispy Roast Chicken (page 155) or Roasted Salmon with Salsa Verde (page 197).

PER SERVING: Calories: 171; Total Fat: 7g; Protein: 8g; Carbohydrates: 21g; Sugars: 3g; Fiber: 7g; Sodium: 565mg

Crispy Parmesan Cups with White Beans and Veggies

Gluten-Free | Vegetarian | Nut-Free | 30 Minutes or Less

Simple meals are really important when changing eating habits, because they allow you to quickly prepare something nourishing before hunger leads to bad choices. This recipe takes just minutes to throw together and is a satisfying vegetable dish bursting with flavor.

CARBS PER SERVING: 24g
SERVINGS: 4 (2 cups each)
PREP TIME: 10 minutes
COOK TIME: 5 minutes

1 cup grated Parmesan cheese, divided

1 (15-ounce) can low-sodium white beans, drained and rinsed

1 cucumber, peeled and finely diced

½ cup finely diced red onion

¼ cup thinly sliced fresh basil

1 garlic clove, minced

½ jalapeño pepper, diced

1 tablespoon extra-virgin olive oil

1 tablespoon balsamic vinegar

¼ teaspoon salt

Freshly ground black pepper

1. Heat a medium nonstick skillet over medium heat. Sprinkle 2 tablespoons of cheese in a thin circle in the center of the pan, flattening it with a spatula.

2. When the cheese melts, use a spatula to flip the cheese and lightly brown the other side.

3. Remove the cheese "pancake" from the pan and place into the cup of a muffin tin, bending it gently with your hands to fit in the muffin cup.

4. Repeat with the remaining cheese until you have 8 cups.

5. In a mixing bowl, combine the beans, cucumber, onion, basil, garlic, jalapeño, olive oil, and vinegar, and season with the salt and pepper.

6. Fill each cup with the bean mixture just before serving.

Substitution tip: If you don't have balsamic vinegar on hand, substitute another light vinegar such as rice vinegar or white wine vinegar.

 Complete the Plate: Add one or two more servings of vegetables to make this a filling and blood sugar-stabilizing meal. I recommend the Roasted Asparagus, Onions, and Red Peppers (page 126) or the Sautéed Spinach and Tomatoes (page 120).

PER SERVING: Calories: 259; Total Fat: 12g; Protein: 15g; Carbohydrates: 24g; Sugars: 4g; Fiber: 8g; Sodium: 551mg

Brussels Sprout, Avocado, and Wild Rice Bowl

Gluten-Free | Vegetarian | Dairy-Free | Nut-Free | 30 Minutes or Less

Dijon mustard is one of the highlights here, and I have to admit, this is my absolute favorite condiment. It enhances the taste of anything you put it on, and there is no added sugar, making it a smart decision for anyone.

CARBS PER SERVING: 18g
SERVINGS: 4
PREP TIME: 15 minutes
COOK TIME: 15 minutes

2 cups sliced
Brussels sprouts

2 teaspoons extra-virgin
olive oil, plus 2 tablespoons

Juice of 1 lemon

1 teaspoon Dijon mustard

1 garlic clove, minced

½ teaspoon salt

¼ teaspoon freshly ground
black pepper

1 cup cooked wild rice

1 cup sliced radishes

1 avocado, sliced

1. Preheat the oven to 400°F. Line a baking sheet with parchment paper.

2. In a medium bowl, toss the Brussels sprouts with 2 teaspoons of olive oil and spread on the prepared baking sheet. Roast for 12 minutes, stirring once, until lightly browned.

3. In a small bowl, mix the remaining 2 tablespoons of olive oil, lemon juice, mustard, garlic, salt, and pepper.

4. In a large bowl, toss the cooked wild rice, radishes, and roasted Brussels sprouts. Drizzle the dressing over the salad and toss.

5. Divide among 4 bowls and top with avocado slices.

Technique tip: On the stove top, add 1 cup wild rice and 4 cups low-sodium broth or water to a medium pot, bring to a boil, cover, and simmer until the grains are cracked open and tender. Depending on the type of wild rice and its age, this can take from 45 to 60 minutes. Freeze extra wild rice in portioned sizes to make using it in recipes quick and easy.

Complete the Plate: This recipe can use another serving of protein as well as another serving of carbs, if desired. Consider adding 4 ounces of grilled tofu or ½ cup shelled edamame, to keep it vegetarian.

PER SERVING: Calories: 178; Total Fat: 11g; Protein: 2g; Carbohydrates: 18g; Sugars: 2g; Fiber: 5g; Sodium: 299mg

Sweet Potato, Chickpea, and Kale Bowl with Creamy Tahini Sauce

Gluten-Free | Vegetarian | Nut-Free | 30 Minutes or Less

This is the ultimate nourishing bowl of goodness during the cold winter months. It is served warm with a creamy and savory tahini sauce. If you haven't tried tahini, a sauce made from toasted sesame seeds, this is a great recipe to start. You might just find yourself adding it to many more dishes. Black beans also work well in this dish. Simply substitute an equal amount of drained and rinsed low-sodium black beans for the chickpeas.

CARBS PER SERVING: 36g
SERVINGS: 2
PREP TIME: 10 minutes
COOK TIME: 15 minutes

FOR THE SAUCE

2 tablespoons plain nonfat Greek yogurt

1 tablespoon tahini

2 tablespoons hemp seeds

1 garlic clove, minced

Pinch salt

Freshly ground black pepper

FOR THE BOWL

1 small sweet potato, peeled and finely diced

1 teaspoon extra-virgin olive oil

1 cup from 1 (15-ounce) can low-sodium chickpeas, drained and rinsed

2 cups baby kale

TO MAKE THE SAUCE

1. In a small bowl, whisk together the yogurt and tahini.

2. Stir in the hemp seeds, garlic, and salt. Season with pepper. Add 2 to 3 tablespoons water to create a creamy yet pourable consistency. Set aside.

TO MAKE THE BOWL

1. Preheat the oven to 425°F. Line a baking sheet with parchment paper.

2. Arrange the sweet potato on the prepared baking sheet and drizzle with the olive oil. Toss. Roast for 10 to 15 minutes, stirring once, until tender and browned.

3. In each of 2 bowls, arrange ½ cup of chickpeas, 1 cup of kale, and half of the cooked sweet potato. Drizzle with half the creamy tahini sauce and serve.

Ingredient tip: If you are new to hemp seeds, let me assure you they are nothing to be skeptical of. While hemp is a variety of the cannabis plant, it is THC free and, in fact, very healthy for us. With a mild, nutty flavor, hemp seeds contain magnesium, zinc, and all essential amino acids, making them a complete, plant-based protein.

 Complete the Plate: This is a complete plate but always has room for additional vegetables if you would like.

PER SERVING: Calories: 322; Total Fat: 14g; Protein: 17g; Carbohydrates: 36g; Sugars: 7g; Fiber: 8g; Sodium: 305mg

Baked Tofu and Mixed Vegetable Bowl

Gluten-Free | Vegetarian | Dairy-Free | Nut-Free | 30 Minutes or Less

Tofu, made from soybeans, is one of the most versatile and affordable protein sources available and is now available in the refrigerated section of most supermarkets. This bowl is a quick and easy meal to throw together for a simple lunch or weeknight dinner. Feel free to swap things up with your favorite vegetables or whatever you have on hand.

CARBS PER SERVING: 22g
SERVINGS: 4
PREP TIME: 10 minutes
COOK TIME: 20 minutes

Nonstick cooking spray

1 (14-ounce) container firm tofu, cut into 1½-inch cubes

2 tablespoons low-sodium gluten-free soy sauce or tamari

1 tablespoon toasted sesame oil

1 teaspoon grated fresh ginger

1 teaspoon honey

2 garlic cloves, minced

2 teaspoons cornstarch

¼ cup water, plus 2 tablespoons

2 teaspoons extra-virgin olive oil

2 cups thinly sliced bok choy

1 cup sliced shiitake mushrooms

1 cup thinly sliced carrots

1 (14-ounce) can baby corn, drained and rinsed

4 scallions, both white and green parts, chopped

1. Preheat the oven to 400°F. Line a baking sheet with parchment paper. Spray the parchment paper with nonstick cooking spray.

2. Place the tofu cubes on the prepared baking sheet and bake for 20 minutes, flipping once, until they are browned.

3. In a small bowl, combine the soy sauce, sesame oil, ginger, honey, and garlic. Stir well to combine.

4. In another small bowl, mix the cornstarch with ¼ cup of water and stir to combine. Add the soy sauce mixture, stir together, and set aside.

5. In a large skillet, heat the oil over medium heat. Add the boy choy, mushrooms, and carrots, and cook for 3 minutes, stirring regularly. Add the remaining 2 tablespoons of water, cover, and steam the vegetables for 3 more minutes until just fork-tender. Add the baby corn.

6. Pour the sauce and cooked tofu into the skillet, and bring to a boil. Reduce the heat and simmer for 1 to 2 minutes until the sauce thickens.

7. Divide the tofu and vegetables among 4 bowls. Top with scallions and serve.

Option tip: Turn up the heat in this dish with a pinch red pepper flakes.

 Complete the Plate: If you prefer, add an extra serving of plant-based protein and high-fiber carbs, such as ½ cup black beans or chickpeas, to each serving.

PER SERVING: Calories: 212; Total Fat: 11g; Protein: 12g; Carbohydrates: 22g; Sugars: 7g; Fiber: 4g; Sodium: 526mg

Mozzarella and Artichoke Stuffed Spaghetti Squash

Gluten-Free | Vegetarian | Nut-Free

These squash bowls got two thumbs up from my Italian in-laws, so I have all the confidence you will love them, too! If you've never tried spaghetti squash, this is the perfect recipe to get you started. Spaghetti squash is a lower-carb pasta substitute that is full of nutrients. Not to mention, it's just a fun vegetable to make, and it's pretty fascinating how the flesh will break off into yummy spaghetti-like strands once it is baked. Buon appetito!

CARBS PER SERVING: 19g
SERVINGS: 4
PREP TIME: 10 minutes
COOK TIME: 45 minutes

1 small spaghetti squash, halved and seeded

½ cup low-fat cottage cheese

¼ cup shredded mozzarella cheese, divided

2 garlic cloves, minced

1 cup artichoke hearts, chopped

1 cup thinly sliced kale

⅛ teaspoon salt

Pinch freshly ground black pepper

1. Preheat the oven to 400°F. Line a baking sheet with parchment paper.

2. Place the cut squash halves on the prepared baking sheet cut-side down, and roast for 30 to 40 minutes, depending on the size and thickness of the squash, until they are fork-tender. Set aside to cool slightly.

3. In a large bowl, mix the cottage cheese, 2 tablespoons of mozzarella cheese, garlic, artichoke hearts, kale, salt, and pepper.

4. Preheat the broiler to high.

5. Using a fork, break apart the flesh of the spaghetti squash into strands, being careful to leave the skin intact. Add the strands to the cheese and vegetable mixture. Toss gently to combine.

6. Divide the mixture between the two hollowed-out squash halves and top with the remaining 2 tablespoons of cheese.

7. Broil for 5 to 7 minutes until browned and heated through.

8. Cut each piece of stuffed squash in half to serve.

Ingredient tip: Look for canned artichoke hearts, not marinated ones, for this recipe. Canned artichoke hearts are typically packed in water, while the marinated ones are packed in oil and spices. If you are unsure, read the label to check the ingredients before buying.

 Complete the Plate: While this recipe has protein, carbs, and veggies, it isn't a stand-alone meal. Consider serving it with your favorite hearty soup, like Tomato and Kale Soup (page 91). Or complete the Italian-inspired meal with Easy Chicken Cacciatore (page 160) or Turkey and Quinoa Caprese Casserole (page 172).

PER SERVING: Calories: 142; Total Fat: 4g; Protein: 9g; Carbohydrates: 19g; Sugars: 10g; Fiber: 4g; Sodium: 312mg

Mushroom Cutlets with Creamy Sauce

Vegetarian

Mushrooms are one of the most versatile vegetables around. And with their natural source of vitamin D, they are a great addition to anyone's diet, especially people with type 2 diabetes. Enjoy these savory and hearty mushroom cutlets as you incorporate more plant-based foods into your diet.

CARBS PER SERVING: 18g

SERVINGS: 4

PREP TIME: 15 minutes

COOK TIME: 20 minutes

FOR THE SAUCE

1 tablespoon extra-virgin olive oil

2 tablespoons whole-wheat flour

1½ cups unsweetened plain almond milk

¼ teaspoon salt

Dash Worcestershire sauce

Pinch cayenne pepper

¼ cup shredded cheddar cheese

TO MAKE THE SAUCE

1. In a medium saucepan, heat the oil over medium heat. Add the flour and stir constantly for about 2 minutes until browned.

2. Slowly whisk in the almond milk and bring to a boil. Reduce the heat to low and simmer for 6 to 8 minutes until the sauce thickens.

3. Season with the salt, Worcestershire sauce, and cayenne. Add the cheese and stir until melted. Turn off the heat and cover to keep warm while you make the cutlets.

FOR THE CUTLETS

2 eggs

2 cups chopped mushrooms

1 cup quick oats

2 scallions, both white and green parts, chopped

¼ cup shredded cheddar cheese

½ teaspoon salt

¼ teaspoon freshly ground black pepper

1 tablespoon extra-virgin olive oil

TO MAKE THE CUTLETS

1. In a large mixing bowl, beat the eggs. Add the mushrooms, oats, scallions, cheese, salt, and pepper. Stir to combine.

2. Using your hands, form the mixture into 8 patties, each about ½ inch thick.

3. In a large skillet, heat the oil over medium-high heat. Cook the patties, in batches if necessary, for 3 minutes per side until crisp and brown.

4. Serve the cutlets warm with sauce drizzled over the top.

Substitution tip: Try a different cheese instead of cheddar for a completely different flavor. Swiss cheese, Havarti, and even a spicy pepper jack can all work here.

 Complete the Plate: While this is a balanced meal, consider adding an additional serving of vegetables and carbs, like Green Salad with Blackberries, Goat Cheese, and Sweet Potatoes (page 103).

PER SERVING: Calories: 261; Total Fat: 17g; Protein: 11g; Carbohydrates: 18g; Sugars: 2g; Fiber: 3g; Sodium: 559mg

Falafel with Creamy Garlic-Yogurt Sauce

Vegetarian | Nut-Free | 30 Minutes or Less

Falafel is often considered a takeout-only menu item, because it seems too complex to cook at home. In fact, it's an easy dish. The balls of falafel are made with chickpeas (sometimes called garbanzo beans), a high-fiber complex carbohydrate that will keep you full and satisfied without spiking blood sugar levels. In this recipe, the falafel are paired with a delicious garlic-yogurt sauce to create a perfect meal.

CARBS PER SERVING: 27g
SERVINGS: 4
PREP TIME: 15 minutes
COOK TIME: 10 minutes

FOR THE SAUCE

¾ cup plain nonfat Greek yogurt

3 garlic cloves, minced

Juice of 1 lemon

1 tablespoon extra-virgin olive oil

¼ teaspoon salt

TO MAKE THE SAUCE

In a small bowl, combine the yogurt, garlic, lemon juice, olive oil, and salt, and mix well. Cover and refrigerate until ready to serve.

TO MAKE THE FALAFEL

1. In a food processor or blender, combine the chickpeas and garlic, and pulse until chopped well but not creamy. Add the flour, parsley, cumin, and salt. Pulse several more times until incorporated.

2. Using your hands, form the mixture into balls, using about 1 tablespoon of mixture for each ball.

3. In a medium skillet, heat 1 teaspoon of canola oil over medium-high heat. Working in batches, add the falafel to the skillet, cooking on each side for 2 to 3 minutes until browned and crisp. Remove the falafel from the skillet, and repeat with the remaining oil and falafel until all are cooked.

FOR THE FALAFEL

1 (15-ounce) can low-sodium
chickpeas, drained
and rinsed

2 garlic cloves,
roughly chopped

2 tablespoons
whole-wheat flour

2 tablespoons chopped
fresh parsley

½ teaspoon ground cumin

¼ teaspoon salt

2 teaspoons canola
oil, divided

8 large lettuce
leaves, chopped

1 cucumber, chopped

1 tomato, diced

4. Divide the lettuce, cucumber, and tomato among 4 plates.

5. Top each plate with 2 falafel and 2 tablespoons of sauce. Serve immediately.

Make-ahead tip: Falafel are best when made directly before serving. However, you can still prep the other ingredients to speed up mealtime. Prepare the lettuce, cucumber, and tomato in advance, and make the garlic-yogurt sauce up to 2 days before using and store in a covered container in the refrigerator.

Complete the Plate: While this recipe is a complete and balanced meal, you might want to add a source of healthy fat, like a few slices of avocado or a drizzle of tahini, and another serving of your favorite vegetables to ensure you are satisfied and energized after your meal.

PER SERVING: Calories: 219; Total Fat: 8g; Protein: 12g; Carbohydrates: 27g; Sugars: 6g; Fiber: 7g; Sodium: 462mg

Lentil Loaf

Gluten-Free | Vegan | Dairy-Free | Nut-Free | Instant Pot Easy

If you are new to lentils, this is the dish to start with. This recipe is one of my absolute favorites. It makes enough to have leftovers throughout the week, so I find myself eating it for both meals and snacks, as it is incredibly filling. You may notice the slightly higher carb content, but do not be concerned; lentils are one of the highest-fiber foods you can eat, making them a healthy choice for anyone, especially those with diabetes. You can also use this same recipe to make veggie lentil burgers by forming the mixture in step 2 into 8 patties. Panfry the patties in 1 tablespoon of olive oil until they're crisp on both sides, about 3 minutes per side.

CARBS PER SERVING: 41g
SERVINGS: 8
PREP TIME: 15 minutes
COOK TIME: 50 minutes

FOR THE GLAZE

¼ cup Low-Carb No-Cook Tomato Ketchup (page 230)

1 tablespoon pure maple syrup

1 tablespoon low-sodium gluten-free soy sauce or tamari

TO MAKE THE GLAZE

In a small bowl, mix together the ketchup, maple syrup, and soy sauce. Set aside.

TO MAKE THE LOAF

1. In an Instant Pot, heat the oil on high. Add the onion, mushrooms, celery, carrot, and garlic, and cook for 2 minutes. Add the lentils, rice, bay leaf, thyme, and 3 cups of water. Cook on high pressure for 10 minutes and release the pressure naturally. Remove the bay leaf.

2. If you don't have an Instant Pot, you can make this on the stove top: Heat the oil in a large pot over medium-high heat. Add the onion, mushrooms, celery, carrot, and garlic, and cook for 2 minutes. Add the lentils, rice, bay leaf, thyme, and 3½ cups of water. Bring to a boil, reduce the heat to low, cover, and simmer for 35 to 45 minutes until the water is absorbed and the lentils and rice are tender. Remove the bay leaf and continue with the recipe.

3. Preheat the oven to 350°F.

4. To the pot, add the hemp seeds, cumin, oregano, paprika, tomato paste, soy sauce, and salt. Stir well.

FOR THE LOAF

1 tablespoon extra-virgin olive oil

1 cup finely chopped onion

1 cup finely chopped mushrooms

1 cup finely chopped celery

1 cup shredded carrot

3 garlic cloves, minced

1½ cups brown lentils

½ cup brown rice

1 bay leaf

½ teaspoon dried thyme

¼ cup hemp seeds

1 teaspoon ground cumin

1 teaspoon dried oregano

1 teaspoon paprika

2 tablespoons tomato paste

2 teaspoons low-sodium gluten-free soy sauce or tamari

½ teaspoon salt

5. Transfer the mixture to a loaf pan, and bake for 20 minutes.

6. Spread the glaze over the loaf, and bake for 20 minutes more. Serve warm.

Make-ahead tip: You can cut prep time by using precooked lentils and brown rice. If you do, preheat the oven first. Heat the oil in a large pot and sauté the vegetables as instructed in step 1. Stir in 3 cups cooked lentils, 1½ cups cooked brown rice, and thyme (omit the bay leaf). Add the hemp seeds, cumin, oregano, paprika, tomato paste, soy sauce, and salt, and stir well. Finish as directed in steps 5 and 6.

Complete the Plate: Complete the plate by adding your favorite vegetable. I love pairing this with Cucumber, Tomato, Avocado Salad (page 101), but you can also add 2 cups of any roasted veggie for a high-fiber, satisfying meal.

PER SERVING: Calories: 258; Total Fat: 5g; Protein: 14g; Carbohydrates: 41g; Sugars: 6g; Fiber: 13g; Sodium: 545mg

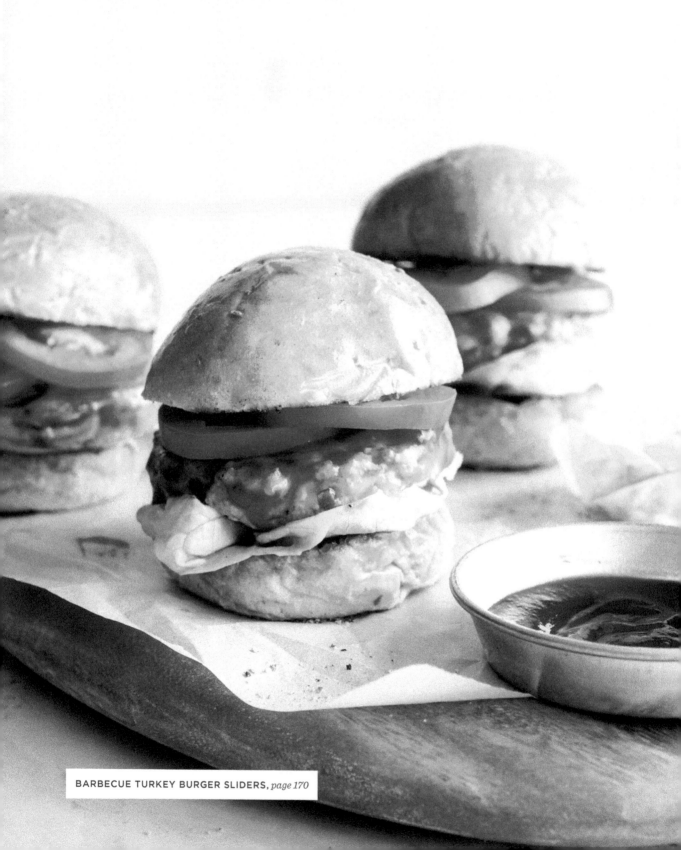

BARBECUE TURKEY BURGER SLIDERS, *page 170*

10

Chicken and Turkey

Easy Coconut Chicken Tenders

Gluten-Free | Dairy-Free | 5-Ingredient | 30 Minutes or Less

If you've never before put coconut and chicken together, I promise you will be pleasantly surprised! The addition of low-carb coconut flour (find it with the grain products in your supermarket) and coconut flakes provides a high-fiber coating that will be nutrient dense, but it won't affect your blood sugar levels. Serve with Low-Carb No-Cook Tomato Ketchup (page 230) to create a combo you'll be sure to love.

CARBS PER SERVING: 9g

SERVINGS: 6
(2 tenders each)

PREP TIME: 10 minutes

COOK TIME: 20 minutes

4 chicken breasts, each cut lengthwise into 3 strips

½ teaspoon salt

¼ teaspoon freshly ground black pepper

½ cup coconut flour

2 eggs, beaten

2 tablespoons unsweetened plain almond milk

1 cup unsweetened coconut flakes

1. Preheat the oven to 400°F. Line a baking sheet with parchment paper.

2. Season the chicken pieces with the salt and pepper.

3. Place the coconut flour in a small bowl. In another bowl, mix the eggs with the almond milk. Spread the coconut flakes on a plate.

4. One by one, roll the chicken pieces in the flour, then dip the floured chicken in the egg mixture and shake off any excess. Roll in the coconut flakes and transfer to the prepared baking sheet.

5. Bake for 15 to 20 minutes, flipping once halfway through, until cooked through and browned.

Option tip: These chicken tenders won't be as browned as traditional deep-fried tenders, so to make a crispier coating, finish the tenders under the broiler for about 1 minute on each side, being careful to watch and prevent burning.

 Complete the Plate: You can serve these chicken tenders with anything. Pair with additional high-fiber carbs and veggies. You could keep it simple and add a small sweet potato with a green salad, or choose a more complex salad like Warm Barley and Squash Salad with Balsamic Vinaigrette (page 107).

PER SERVING: Calories: 216; Total Fat: 13g; Protein: 20g; Carbohydrates: 9g; Sugars: 2g; Fiber: 6g; Sodium: 346mg

Chicken Caesar Salad

Gluten-Free | Nut-Free | 30 Minutes or Less

You can make this classic salad at home, and it will taste just as amazing as one you would order at your favorite restaurant. I love adding this to my menu during the spring and summer months because it is simple and refreshing. It's a perfect meal to serve when you have a nice summer dinner party with your friends or family.

CARBS PER SERVING: 6g
SERVINGS: 2
PREP TIME: 10 minutes
COOK TIME: 15 minutes

1 garlic clove

½ teaspoon anchovy paste

Juice of ½ lemon

2 tablespoons extra-virgin olive oil

1 (8-ounce) boneless, skinless chicken breast

¼ teaspoon salt

Freshly ground black pepper

2 romaine lettuce hearts, cored and chopped

1 red bell pepper, seeded and cut into thin strips

¼ cup grated Parmesan cheese

1. Preheat the broiler to high.

2. In a blender jar, combine the garlic, anchovy paste, lemon juice, and olive oil. Process until smooth and set aside.

3. Cut the chicken breast lengthwise into two even cutlets of similar thickness. Season the chicken with the salt and pepper, and place on a baking sheet.

4. Broil the chicken for 5 to 7 minutes on each side until cooked through and browned. Cut into thin strips.

5. In a medium mixing bowl, toss the lettuce, bell pepper, and cheese. Add the dressing and toss to coat. Divide the salad between 2 plates and top with the chicken.

Option tip: While a traditional Caesar salad includes croutons, I've left them out here to keep the carb count low. However, feel free to add any nonstarchy vegetables to the salad to make it your own. Cucumbers, radishes, artichoke hearts, roasted asparagus, and shredded carrots all work well in this simple Caesar.

Complete the Plate: You can add carbs to this meal, as desired. It can be as simple as a small sweet potato or whole fruit, or you can serve it alongside a Red Pepper, Goat Cheese, and Arugula Open-Faced Grilled Sandwich (page 113).

PER SERVING: Calories: 292; Total Fat: 18g; Protein: 28g; Carbohydrates: 6g; Sugars: 3g; Fiber: 2g; Sodium: 706mg

Spice-Rubbed Crispy Roast Chicken

Gluten-Free | Dairy-Free | Nut-Free

Everyone needs a quick and easy go-to chicken recipe, and this is mine. The combination of five of my favorite spices with just a pinch salt is the perfect blend, which can be used on anything you like, from proteins to veggies to your favorite homemade soups.

CARBS PER SERVING: 1g
SERVINGS: 6
PREP TIME: 10 minutes
COOK TIME: 35 minutes

1 teaspoon ground paprika

1 teaspoon garlic powder

½ teaspoon ground coriander

½ teaspoon ground cumin

½ teaspoon salt

¼ teaspoon ground cayenne pepper

6 chicken legs

1 teaspoon extra-virgin olive oil

1. Preheat the oven to 400°F.

2. In a small bowl, combine the paprika, garlic powder, coriander, cumin, salt, and cayenne pepper. Rub the chicken legs all over with the spices.

3. In an ovenproof skillet, heat the oil over medium heat. Sear the chicken for 8 to 10 minutes on each side until the skin browns and becomes crisp.

4. Transfer the skillet to the oven and continue to cook for 10 to 15 minutes until the chicken is cooked through and its juices run clear.

Substitution tip: Skin-on, bone-in chicken breasts work great with this rub, as well, and are leaner but take longer to cook. Plan on 2 servings per chicken breast. Sear only the skin side, and increase the baking time to 45 minutes, flipping once halfway through.

 Complete the Plate: This protein-rich dish still needs veggies and carbohydrates. Add your favorite veggie-loaded soup, like Curried Carrot Soup (page 94), and/or Warm Barley and Squash Salad with Balsamic Vinaigrette (page 107).

PER SERVING: Calories: 276; Total Fat: 16g; Protein: 30g; Carbohydrates: 1g; Sugars: 0g; Fiber: 0g; Sodium: 256mg

Saffron-Spiced Chicken Breasts

Gluten-Free | Nut-Free

Saffron is an ancient orange spice that has been found to have several health benefits. It provides a subtle, sweet flavor that is very recognizable. Find it at your local Middle Eastern specialty store or gourmet grocery store or, of course, on Amazon!

CARBS PER SERVING: 3g
SERVINGS: 4
PREP TIME: 10 minutes, plus 1 hour to marinate
COOK TIME: 10 minutes

Pinch saffron (3 or 4 threads)

½ cup plain nonfat yogurt

2 tablespoons water

½ onion, chopped

3 garlic cloves, minced

2 tablespoons chopped fresh cilantro

Juice of ½ lemon

½ teaspoon salt

1 pound boneless, skinless chicken breasts, cut into 2-inch strips

1 tablespoon extra-virgin olive oil

1. In a blender jar, combine the saffron, yogurt, water, onion, garlic, cilantro, lemon juice, and salt. Pulse to blend.

2. In a large mixing bowl, combine the chicken and the yogurt sauce, and stir to coat. Cover and refrigerate for at least 1 hour or up to overnight.

3. In a large skillet, heat the oil over medium heat. Add the chicken pieces, shaking off any excess marinade. Discard the marinade. Cook the chicken pieces on each side for 5 minutes, flipping once, until cooked through and golden brown.

Substitution tip: If you don't have saffron, substitute ½ teaspoon of turmeric for a similar color and flavor.

 Complete the Plate: Serve with your favorite salad or nonstarchy vegetable side along with a starchy vegetable or grain side. I suggest adding Green Salad with Blackberries, Goat Cheese, and Sweet Potatoes (page 103) or a simple side salad and up to ⅔ cup brown or wild rice.

PER SERVING: Calories: 155; Total Fat: 5g; Protein: 26g; Carbohydrates: 3g; Sugars: 1g; Fiber: 0g; Sodium: 501mg

Sesame-Ginger Chicken Soba

Gluten-Free | Dairy-Free | Nut-Free | 30 Minutes or Less

Soba noodles are made from buckwheat, so they are naturally gluten free, and are loaded with nutrition. While they aren't much lower in carbs than regular pasta, they are higher in both fiber and protein, making them lower on the glycemic index and therefore a better choice for your blood sugar levels.

CARBS PER SERVING: 35g
SERVINGS: 6
PREP TIME: 10 minutes
COOK TIME: 15 minutes

8 ounces soba noodles

2 boneless, skinless chicken breasts, halved lengthwise

¼ cup tahini

2 tablespoons rice vinegar

1 tablespoon reduced-sodium gluten-free soy sauce or tamari

1 teaspoon toasted sesame oil

1 (1-inch) piece fresh ginger, finely grated

⅓ cup water

1 large cucumber, seeded and diced

1 scallions bunch, green parts only, cut into 1-inch segments

1 tablespoon sesame seeds

1. Preheat the broiler to high.

2. Bring a large pot of water to a boil. Add the noodles and cook until tender, according to the package directions. Drain and rinse the noodles in cool water.

3. On a baking sheet, arrange the chicken in a single layer. Broil for 5 to 7 minutes on each side, depending on the thickness, until the chicken is cooked through and its juices run clear. Use two forks to shred the chicken.

4. In a small bowl, combine the tahini, rice vinegar, soy sauce, sesame oil, ginger, and water. Whisk to combine.

5. In a large bowl, toss the shredded chicken, noodles, cucumber, and scallions. Pour the tahini sauce over the noodles and toss to combine. Served sprinkled with the sesame seeds.

Option tip: To make sure this recipe is gluten free, look for 100 percent buckwheat soba noodles. Buckwheat is a plant that is cultivated for its seeds, which are similar to a grain but are actually not. Buckwheat is not related to wheat at all.

Complete the Plate: Add at least 2 servings of non-starchy vegetables like Roasted Lemon and Garlic Broccoli (page 122) or Garlicky Cabbage and Collard Greens (page 121).

PER SERVING: Calories: 251; Total Fat: 8g; Protein: 16g; Carbohydrates: 35g; Sugars: 2g; Fiber: 2g; Sodium: 482mg

Quick Weeknight Chicken Parmesan

Gluten-Free

Let's be honest, cooking dinner every night of the week is not a realistic option for most of us. I'm a big fan of the "cook once, eat twice" method to make meals go further. This quick chicken Parmesan is satisfying and easy enough to add to your weekly rotation. Make your veggies while it is cooking and you will have dinner on the table in a hurry.

CARBS PER SERVING: 21g
SERVINGS: 4
PREP TIME: 10 minutes
COOK TIME: 30 minutes

½ cup rolled oats

¼ teaspoon freshly ground black pepper

1 large egg

2 tablespoons unsweetened plain almond milk

¼ cup grated Parmesan cheese

¼ cup gluten-free bread crumbs

1 pound boneless, skinless chicken breast, cut lengthwise into 4 cutlets

1 cup Quick Tomato Marinara (page 231), divided

¼ cup shredded mozzarella cheese

1. Preheat the oven to 400°F.

2. In a blender or food processor, process the oats until they resemble flour. Transfer to a medium bowl and mix with the pepper.

3. In another medium bowl, combine the egg and almond milk and lightly beat.

4. On a plate, mix the Parmesan cheese with the bread crumbs.

5. One at a time, roll the chicken pieces in the oat flour, dip in the egg mixture, and roll in the Parmesan-bread crumb mixture. Arrange the chicken pieces in a single layer in a baking dish.

6. Bake for 25 minutes until the chicken is cooked through and the coating is browned.

7. Spoon half of the marinara over the chicken, along with 1 tablespoon of cheese over each piece. Bake 5 more minutes until the cheese is melted.

8. Serve topped with the remaining marinara sauce.

Substitution tip: If you want something lighter, try using a large portobello mushroom rather than chicken. Lightly wet the mushroom before rolling in the flour, and continue with the recipe as written for a vegetarian take on the original.

 Complete the Plate: Add your favorite vegetables to complete the plate. I enjoy adding Roasted Asparagus, Onions, and Red Peppers (page 126) or Sautéed Spinach and Tomatoes (page 120).

PER SERVING: Calories: 295; Total Fat: 11g; Protein: 33g; Carbohydrates: 18g; Sugars: 2g; Fiber: 2g; Sodium: 612mg

Easy Chicken Cacciatore

Gluten-Free | Dairy-Free | Nut-Free

Chicken cacciatore is a dish I always recommend my clients look for at their favorite Italian restaurant. It's naturally low in carbs and full of freshness from the plentiful herbs, spices, and vegetables it contains. Make this traditional version in the comfort of your own home, and you will have enough for leftovers the next day.

CARBS PER SERVING: 11g
SERVINGS: 6
PREP TIME: 10 minutes
COOK TIME: 45 minutes

3 teaspoons extra-virgin olive oil, divided

6 chicken legs

8 ounces brown mushrooms

1 large onion, sliced

1 red bell pepper, seeded and cut into strips

3 garlic cloves, minced

½ cup dry red wine

1 (28-ounce) can whole tomatoes, drained

1 thyme sprig

1 rosemary sprig

½ teaspoon salt

¼ teaspoon freshly ground black pepper

¼ cup water

1. Preheat the oven to 350°F.

2. In a Dutch oven (or any oven-safe covered pot), heat 2 teaspoons of oil over medium-high heat. Sear the chicken on all sides until browned. Remove and set aside.

3. Heat the remaining 1 teaspoon of oil in the Dutch oven and sauté the mushrooms for 3 to 5 minutes until they brown and begin to release their water. Add the onion, bell pepper, and garlic, and mix together with the mushrooms. Cook an additional 3 to 5 minutes until the onion begins to soften.

4. Add the red wine and deglaze the pot. Bring to a simmer. Add the tomatoes, breaking them into pieces with a spoon. Add the thyme, rosemary, salt, and pepper to the pot and mix well.

5. Add the water, then nestle the cooked chicken, along with any juices that have accumulated, in the vegetables.

6. Transfer the pot to the oven. Cook for 30 minutes until the chicken is cooked through and its juices run clear. Remove the thyme and rosemary sprigs and serve.

Substitution tip: If you don't have fresh herbs, use ½ teaspoon each of dried thyme and rosemary.

 Complete the Plate: Complete this Italian plate by pairing with Crispy Parmesan Cups with White Beans and Veggies (page 136) or Three Bean and Basil Salad (page 105).

PER SERVING: Calories: 257; Total Fat: 11g; Protein: 28g; Carbohydrates: 11g; Sugars: 6g; Fiber: 2g; Sodium: 398mg

Peanut Chicken Satay

Gluten-Free

These Indonesian-inspired chicken skewers are perfect for any occasion. From Saturday evening dinner parties to Sunday brunches, they have proven to be both toddler and husband approved in my house, so I know they will be a hit with your family, as well.

CARBS PER SERVING: 14g

SERVINGS: 8

PREP TIME: 20 minutes, plus 2 hours to marinate

COOK TIME: 10 minutes

FOR THE PEANUT SAUCE

1 cup natural peanut butter

2 tablespoons low-sodium tamari or gluten-free soy sauce

1 teaspoon red chili paste

1 tablespoon honey

Juice of 2 limes

½ cup hot water

TO MAKE THE PEANUT SAUCE

In a medium mixing bowl, combine the peanut butter, tamari, chili paste, honey, lime juice, and hot water. Mix until smooth. Set aside.

TO MAKE THE CHICKEN

1. In a large mixing bowl, combine the chicken, yogurt, garlic, ginger, onion, coriander, cumin, and salt, and mix well.

2. Cover and marinate in the refrigerator for at least 2 hours.

3. Thread the chicken pieces onto bamboo skewers.

4. In a grill pan or large skillet, heat the oil. Cook the skewers for 3 to 5 minutes on each side until the pieces are cooked through.

FOR THE CHICKEN

2 pounds boneless, skinless chicken thighs, trimmed of fat and cut into 1-inch pieces

½ cup plain nonfat Greek yogurt

2 garlic cloves, minced

1 teaspoon minced fresh ginger

½ onion, coarsely chopped

1½ teaspoons ground coriander

2 teaspoons ground cumin

½ teaspoon salt

1 teaspoon extra-virgin olive oil

Lettuce leaves, for serving

5. Remove the chicken from the skewers and place a few pieces on each lettuce leaf. Drizzle with the peanut sauce and serve.

Technique tip: Alternatively, cook the skewers over a medium hot barbecue grill for 3 to 5 minutes per side until cooked through.

Complete the Plate: Add at least 1 to 2 cups of vegetables to this meal. I love Roasted Asparagus, Onions, and Red Peppers (page 126) or simply roasting whatever veggies I have on hand. You can also add a ½ cup serving of quinoa or brown rice.

PER SERVING: Calories: 386; Total Fat: 26g; Protein: 30g; Carbohydrates: 14g; Sugars: 6g; Fiber: 2g; Sodium: 442mg

Teriyaki Turkey Meatballs

Gluten-Free | Dairy-Free | Nut-Free

These simple baked meatballs are a tasty, high-protein addition to any meal or snack. With powerful nutrients coming from the garlic and ginger, you can rest assured these will be healthy for you and safe for your blood sugar levels. Freeze any extra meatballs so you have a quick option when you need fast, low-carb food.

CARBS PER SERVING: 5g

SERVINGS: 6

(4 meatballs each)

PREP TIME: 20 minutes

COOK TIME: 20 minutes

1 pound lean ground turkey

¼ cup finely chopped scallions, both white and green parts

1 egg

2 garlic cloves, minced

1 teaspoon grated fresh ginger

2 tablespoons reduced-sodium tamari or gluten-free soy sauce

1 tablespoon honey

2 teaspoons mirin

1 teaspoon toasted sesame oil

1. Preheat the oven to 400°F. Line a baking sheet with parchment paper.

2. In a large mixing bowl, combine the turkey, scallions, egg, garlic, ginger, tamari, honey, mirin, and sesame oil. Mix well.

3. Using your hands, form the meat mixture into balls about the size of a tablespoon. Arrange on the prepared baking sheet.

4. Bake for 10 minutes, flip with a spatula, and continue baking for an additional 10 minutes until the meatballs are cooked through.

Ingredient tip: Teriyaki is a Japanese cooking technique where foods are broiled or grilled using a glaze that combines soy sauce, mirin (a low-alcohol rice wine used for cooking), and sugar. In this lighter version, honey replaces sugar, and the soy-mirin-honey is packed into the meatballs instead of glazing them, giving you a flavorful meatball that is light and delicious while still loaded with teriyaki flavor.

 Complete the Plate: **Serve with your favorite vegetables and 1 to 2 servings of carbohydrates. Recommended choices include Green Salad with Blackberries, Goat Cheese, and Sweet Potatoes (page 103) and Tomato and Kale Soup (page 91).**

PER SERVING: Calories: 153; Total Fat: 8g; Protein: 16g; Carbohydrates: 5g; Sugars: 4g; Fiber: 0g; Sodium: 270mg

Turkey Meatloaf Muffins

Gluten-Free | Dairy-Free | Nut-Free

Individual servings of meatloaf are one of the easiest things to add to your meal-prepping plan. Use these as a snack or as part of a main meal. I love the oat flour addition, and I hope you will think of using this nutrient-rich flour alternative in other foods you commonly make, such as muffins and pancakes, or as toppings to baked dishes. You can actually substitute oat flour one-for-one for wheat flour.

CARBS PER SERVING: 4g

SERVINGS: 12

(2 muffins each)

PREP TIME: 10 minutes

COOK TIME: 35 minutes

Nonstick cooking spray

½ cup old-fashioned oats

1 pound lean ground turkey

½ cup finely chopped onion

1 red bell pepper, seeded and finely chopped

2 eggs

3 garlic cloves, minced

1 teaspoon salt

½ teaspoon freshly ground black pepper

1. Preheat the oven to 375°F. Lightly spray a 12-cup muffin tin with nonstick cooking spray.

2. In a blender, process the oats until they become flour.

3. In a large mixing bowl, combine the oat flour, turkey, onion, bell pepper, eggs, and garlic. Mix well and season with the salt and pepper.

4. Using an ice cream scoop, transfer a ¼-cup portion of the meat mixture to each muffin cup.

5. Bake for 30 to 35 minutes until the muffins are cooked through.

6. Slide a knife along the outside of each cup to loosen the muffins and remove. Serve warm.

◆▸

Option tip: If you would like a glaze on your meatloaf, mix ¼ cup Low-Carb No-Cook Tomato Ketchup (page 230) with 1 tablespoon pure maple syrup and 1 teaspoon gluten-free soy sauce and spread it on the turkey muffins during the last 5 minutes of cooking.

 Complete the Plate: Make it a meal by adding your favorite soup and salad. I love Cabbage Slaw Salad (page 102) and Tomato and Kale Soup (page 91) with this dish.

PER SERVING: Calories: 88; Total Fat: 4g; Protein: 9g; Carbohydrates: 4g; Sugars: 1g; Fiber: 1g; Sodium: 203mg

Mushroom-Sage Stuffed Turkey Breast

Gluten-Free | 5-Ingredient

Savory mushrooms come together with fresh sage in this comforting stuffed turkey breast. Mushrooms are one of the few dietary sources of vitamin D, a nutrient of concern for those with diabetes, so this is a tasty way to get some important vitamins. I hope this dish will remind you that turkey isn't just for November but can be enjoyed year-round.

CARBS PER SERVING: 2g

SERVINGS: 8

PREP TIME: 10 minutes

COOK TIME: 1 hour, 5 minutes

2 tablespoons extra-virgin olive oil, divided

8 ounces brown mushrooms, finely chopped

2 garlic cloves, minced

½ teaspoon salt, divided

¼ teaspoon freshly ground black pepper, divided

2 tablespoons chopped fresh sage

1 boneless, skinless turkey breast (about 3 pounds), butterflied

1. Preheat the oven to 375°F.

2. In a large skillet, heat 1 tablespoon of oil over medium heat. Add the mushrooms and cook for 4 to 5 minutes, stirring regularly, until most of the liquid has evaporated from the pan. Add the garlic, ¼ teaspoon of salt, and ⅛ teaspoon of pepper, and continue to cook for an additional minute. Add the sage to the pan, cook for 1 minute, and remove the pan from the heat.

3. On a clean work surface, lay the turkey breast flat. Use a kitchen mallet to pound the breast to an even 1-inch thickness throughout.

4. Spread the mushroom-sage mixture on the turkey breast, leaving a 1-inch border around the edges. Roll the breast tightly into a log.

5. Using kitchen twine, tie the breast two or three times around to hold it together. Rub the remaining 1 tablespoon of oil over the turkey breast. Season with the remaining ¼ teaspoon of salt and ⅛ teaspoon of pepper.

6. Transfer to a roasting pan and roast for 50 to 60 minutes, until the juices run clear, the meat is cooked through, and the internal temperature reaches 180°F.

7. Let rest for 5 minutes. Cut off the twine, slice, and serve.

Technique tip: To butterfly a turkey breast, start with a boneless, skinless breast. If the turkey breast came rolled in netting or tied, remove the netting as well as any pop-up thermometer. Unroll the turkey breast, and if any skin remains, use a knife to cut it away from the meat. Lay the turkey breast so the side that used to have skin is facing down. Beginning at the narrowest side, hold the knife parallel to the cutting board and make a horizontal cut through the center of the breast, stopping about an inch before separating the two pieces. Open the breast and it should fold out like a book. It is now ready to be pounded and stuffed.

Complete the Plate: Keep it simple and add 1 to 2 cups of your favorite veggies alongside 1 to 2 servings of healthy carbs such as a small sweet potato, ½ cup of quinoa, or Roasted Delicata Squash (page 125).

PER SERVING: Calories: 232; Total Fat: 6g; Protein: 41g; Carbohydrates: 2g; Sugars: 0g; Fiber: 0g; Sodium: 320mg

Turkey Chili

Gluten-Free · Nut-Free

Chili has always been one of my favorite comfort foods, and many people don't realize it can be one of the healthiest comfort foods, as well! This version is lower in sodium yet still has tons of flavor. It's a great source of fiber with about 8 grams per serving, making it a safe meal for those with diabetes, as it will not spike blood sugar levels.

CARBS PER SERVING: 27g
SERVINGS: 6
PREP TIME: 15 minutes
COOK TIME: 30 minutes

1 tablespoon extra-virgin olive oil

1 pound lean ground turkey

1 large onion, diced

3 garlic cloves, minced

1 red bell pepper, seeded and diced

1 cup chopped celery

2 tablespoons chili powder

1 tablespoon ground cumin

1 (28-ounce) can reduced-salt diced tomatoes

1 (15-ounce) can low-sodium kidney beans, drained and rinsed

2 cups low-sodium chicken broth

½ teaspoon salt

Shredded cheddar cheese, for serving (optional)

1. In a large pot, heat the oil over medium heat. Add the turkey, onion, and garlic, and cook, stirring regularly, until the turkey is cooked through.

2. Add the bell pepper, celery, chili powder, and cumin. Stir well and continue to cook for 1 minute.

3. Add the tomatoes with their liquid, kidney beans, and chicken broth. Bring to a boil, reduce the heat to low, and simmer for 20 minutes.

4. Season with the salt and serve topped with cheese (if using).

Option tip: If you like a little heat in your chili, add 1 seeded and diced serrano or jalapeño pepper in step 2 along with the bell pepper, celery, and spices.

Complete the Plate: While this is a full plate, I recommend adding a dollop of 2 percent Greek yogurt and a few slices of avocado for some additional protein and healthy fat. And as always, you can add more vegetables if you would like.

PER SERVING: Calories: 276; Total Fat: 10g; Protein: 23g; Carbohydrates: 27g; Sugars: 7g; Fiber: 8g; Sodium: 556mg

Barbecue Turkey Burger Sliders

Dairy-Free | Nut-Free | 30 Minutes or Less

Sliders have always been a family favorite in our household, and with a few improvements, we can add more fiber and nutrients to them, making them a better option for anyone. This is the perfect addition to your next family gathering or celebration. I hope you'll enjoy them on a warm summer day while relaxing with those you love the most as you rest assured these won't spike your blood sugar levels.

CARBS PER SERVING: 26g

SERVINGS: 4

PREP TIME: 15 minutes

COOK TIME: 15 minutes

FOR THE SAUCE

½ cup Low-Carb No-Cook Tomato Ketchup (page 230)

2 tablespoons apple cider vinegar

1 tablespoon pure maple syrup

½ teaspoon freshly ground black pepper

½ teaspoon onion powder

Juice of ½ lemon

½ teaspoon Worcestershire sauce

Freshly ground white pepper

TO MAKE THE SAUCE

1. In a small saucepan, combine the ketchup, vinegar, maple syrup, black pepper, onion powder, lemon juice, Worcestershire sauce, and white pepper, and bring to a simmer over medium heat.

2. Simmer for about 5 minutes until the sauce is thickened. Set aside.

FOR THE BURGERS

8 ounces lean ground turkey

1 celery stalk, finely chopped

1 scallion, both white and green parts, finely chopped

4 whole-wheat dinner rolls, split

4 lettuce leaves

4 tomato slices

TO MAKE THE BURGERS

1. In a mixing bowl, combine the turkey, celery, and scallion, and stir well to combine. Form the turkey mixture into 4 small patties.

2. In a grill pan or a cast iron pan over medium-high heat, brown the burgers for about 3 minutes on each side. Using a pastry brush, glaze the tops of the burgers with the barbecue sauce, then flip, and spread sauce on the opposite side. Continue to cook until the juices run clear.

3. Open the dinner rolls and place one burger in each. Top with lettuce and tomato, and serve.

Substitution tip: You can use a low-sugar store-bought barbecue sauce in place of homemade, if you already have one on hand. And if you are looking to reduce the carbs further, you can always skip the bun, which is where most of the carbs in this recipe come from.

 Complete the Plate: Serve alongside your favorite veggies. These sliders pair perfectly with Garlicky Cabbage and Collard Greens (page 121) or Cabbage Slaw Salad (page 102).

PER SERVING: Calories: 213; Total Fat: 7g; Protein: 15g; Carbohydrates: 26g; Sugars: 11g; Fiber: 4g; Sodium: 276mg

Turkey and Quinoa Caprese Casserole

Gluten-Free | Nut-Free

One-dish meals are my favorite, and this Italian-inspired casserole is no exception. It combines protein-rich quinoa and turkey with fresh vegetables and herbs to provide a well-balanced meal. It's convenient to make this casserole on the weekend and delicious enough to eat it throughout your week.

CARBS PER SERVING: 17g
SERVINGS: 8
PREP TIME: 10 minutes
COOK TIME: 35 minutes

⅔ cup quinoa

1⅓ cups water

Nonstick cooking spray

2 teaspoons extra-virgin olive oil

1 pound lean ground turkey

¼ cup chopped red onion

½ teaspoon salt

1 (15-ounce can) fire-roasted tomatoes, drained

4 cups spinach leaves, finely sliced

3 garlic cloves, minced

¼ cup sliced fresh basil

¼ cup chicken or vegetable broth

2 large ripe tomatoes, sliced

4 ounces mozzarella cheese, thinly sliced

1. In a small pot, combine the quinoa and water. Bring to a boil, reduce the heat, cover, and simmer for 10 minutes. Turn off the heat, and let the quinoa sit for 5 minutes to absorb any remaining water.

2. Preheat the oven to 400°F. Spray a baking dish with non-stick cooking spray.

3. In a large skillet, heat the oil over medium heat. Add the turkey, onion, and salt. Cook until the turkey is cooked through and crumbled.

4. Add the tomatoes, spinach, garlic, and basil. Stir in the broth and cooked quinoa. Transfer the mixture to the prepared baking dish. Arrange the tomato and cheese slices on top.

5. Bake for 15 minutes until the cheese is melted and the tomatoes are softened. Serve.

Option tip: Substitute ground chicken, pork, or beef for an alternative to this dish. If you're using beef, omit the oil, and drain as much grease from the pan as possible after cooking the meat before proceeding to step 4.

 Complete the Plate: While this recipe will complete the plate, it's not a stand-alone meal. Feel free to enjoy 2 servings of this dish or serve with an additional side of healthy carbs, like Roasted Delicata Squash (page 125), or a simple green salad with Easy Italian Dressing (page 238).

PER SERVING: Calories: 218; Total Fat: 9g; Protein: 18g; Carbohydrates: 17g; Sugars: 3g; Fiber: 3g; Sodium: 340mg

Turkey Divan Casserole

This dish was inspired by the always-present casserole recipes in the many Southern cookbooks I own. They are some of the cookbooks I cherish most, as many of them were passed down to me from close family members or given to me as gifts. When I'm in need of inspiration, I always go back to them. This comforting casserole is enhanced to provide more nutritional benefits, without all the carbs. I hope you will find it as nourishing for the soul and body as I do. Enjoy!

CARBS PER SERVING: 9g

SERVINGS: 6

PREP TIME: 10 minutes

COOK TIME: 50 minutes

Nonstick cooking spray

3 teaspoons extra-virgin olive oil, divided

1 pound turkey cutlets

Pinch salt

¼ teaspoon freshly ground black pepper, divided

¼ cup chopped onion

2 garlic cloves, minced

2 tablespoons whole-wheat flour

1 cup unsweetened plain almond milk

1 cup low-sodium chicken broth

½ cup shredded Swiss cheese, divided

½ teaspoon dried thyme

4 cups chopped broccoli

¼ cup coarsely ground almonds

1. Preheat the oven to 375°F. Spray a baking dish with non-stick cooking spray.

2. In a skillet, heat 1 teaspoon of oil over medium heat. Season the turkey with the salt and ⅛ teaspoon of pepper. Sauté the turkey cutlets for 5 to 7 minutes on each side until cooked through. Transfer to a cutting board, cool briefly, and cut into bite-size pieces.

3. In the same pan, heat the remaining 2 teaspoons of oil over medium-high heat. Sauté the onion for 3 minutes until it begins to soften. Add the garlic and continue cooking for another minute.

4. Stir in the flour and mix well. Whisk in the almond milk, broth, and remaining ⅛ teaspoon of pepper, and continue whisking until smooth. Add ¼ cup of cheese and the thyme, and continue stirring until the cheese is melted.

5. In the prepared baking dish, arrange the broccoli on the bottom. Cover with half the sauce. Place the turkey pieces on top of the broccoli, and cover with the remaining sauce. Sprinkle with the remaining ¼ cup of cheese and the ground almonds.

6. Bake for 35 minutes until the sauce is bubbly and the top is browned.

Option tip: For a sauce with some kick, add ¼ teaspoon cayenne pepper to the cheese sauce in step 4.

 Complete the Plate: You can add another 1 or 2 servings of carbs to this meal and, as always, additional vegetables. You may consider Roasted Delicata Squash (page 125) or Cucumber, Tomato, and Avocado Salad (page 101).

PER SERVING: Calories: 207; Total Fat: 8g; Protein: 25g; Carbohydrates: 9g; Sugars: 2g; Fiber: 3g; Sodium: 128mg

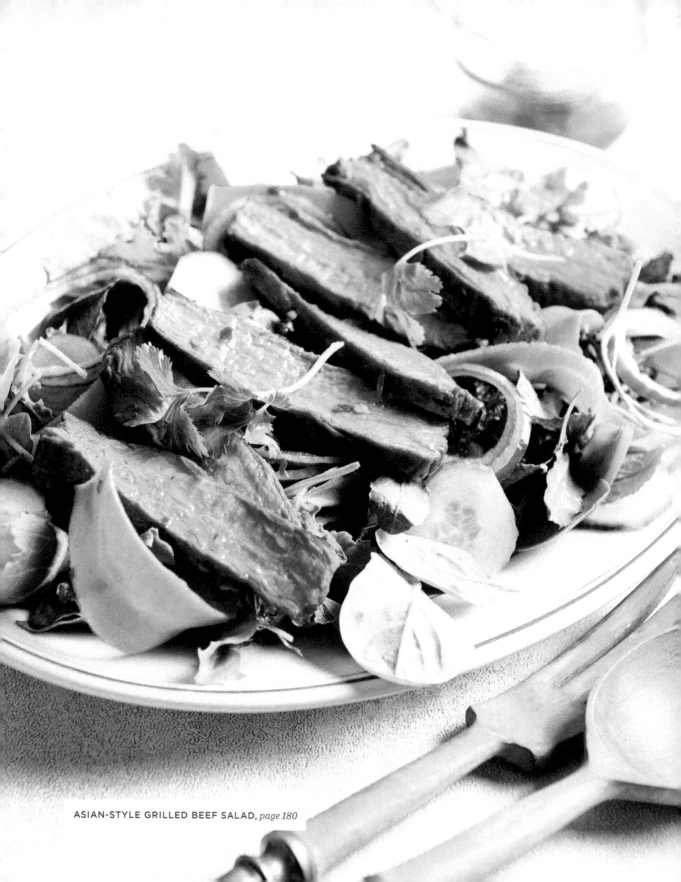

ASIAN-STYLE GRILLED BEEF SALAD, *page 180*

11
Beef, Pork, and Lamb

Bunless Sloppy Joes

Gluten-Free | Dairy-Free | Nut-Free

Sloppy Joes are one of the most classic American sandwiches of all time and are very popular for a good reason: They taste amazing! This healthier version still keeps the flavor we have all grown to love, while skipping the bun and replacing it with a baked sweet potato—a more nutritious starch that will add an exciting new flavor spin to this famous dish.

CARBS PER SERVING: 34g
SERVINGS: 6
PREP TIME: 15 minutes
COOK TIME: 40 minutes

6 small sweet potatoes
1 pound lean ground beef
1 onion, finely chopped
1 carrot, finely chopped
¼ cup finely chopped mushrooms
¼ cup finely chopped red bell pepper
3 garlic cloves, minced
2 teaspoons Worcestershire sauce
1 tablespoon white wine vinegar
1 (15-ounce) can low-sodium tomato sauce
2 tablespoons tomato paste

1. Preheat the oven to 400°F.

2. Place the sweet potatoes in a single layer in a baking dish. Bake for 25 to 40 minutes, depending on the size, until they are soft and cooked through.

3. While the sweet potatoes are baking, in a large skillet, cook the beef over medium heat until it's browned, breaking it apart into small pieces as you stir.

4. Add the onion, carrot, mushrooms, bell pepper, and garlic, and sauté briefly for 1 minute.

5. Stir in the Worcestershire sauce, vinegar, tomato sauce, and tomato paste. Bring to a simmer, reduce the heat, and cook for 5 minutes for the flavors to meld.

6. Scoop ½ cup of the meat mixture on top of each baked potato and serve.

Technique tip: If you want to shave some time off prep, chop the vegetables in a food processor.

 Complete the Plate: While this meal does create a balanced plate, you can always add some additional vegetables. I love Cabbage Slaw Salad (page 102) with this dish.

PER SERVING: Calories: 372; Total Fat: 19g; Protein: 16g; Carbohydrates: 34g; Sugars: 13g; Fiber: 6g; Sodium: 161mg

Easy Beef Curry

Gluten-Free | Dairy-Free | Nut-Free | 30 Minutes or Less

Using a quality lean meat speeds up cooking time, compared with the more traditional long-simmered cuts used in a beef curry. I recommend grass-fed meats because they have a higher ratio of good-for-you omega-3 fatty acids and contain more antioxidant vitamins than beef raised on commercial feed. Enjoy the magical blend of herbs and spices that creates a savory and crave-worthy curry while also making use of the health-promoting benefits of some of mother nature's oldest "medicines," found in these spices.

CARBS PER SERVING: 3g

SERVINGS: 6

PREP TIME: 15 minutes

COOK TIME: 10 minutes

1 tablespoon extra-virgin olive oil

1 small onion, thinly sliced

2 teaspoons minced fresh ginger

3 garlic cloves, minced

2 teaspoons ground coriander

1 teaspoon ground cumin

1 jalapeño or serrano pepper, slit lengthwise but not all the way through

¼ teaspoon ground turmeric

¼ teaspoon salt

1 pound grass-fed sirloin tip steak, top round steak, or top sirloin steak, cut into bite-size pieces

2 tablespoons chopped fresh cilantro

1. In a large skillet, heat the oil over medium high.

2. Add the onion, and cook for 3 to 5 minutes until browned and softened. Add the ginger and garlic, stirring continuously until fragrant, about 30 seconds.

3. In a small bowl, mix the coriander, cumin, jalapeño, turmeric, and salt. Add the spice mixture to the skillet and stir continuously for 1 minute. Deglaze the skillet with about ¼ cup of water.

4. Add the beef and stir continuously for about 5 minutes until well-browned yet still medium rare. Remove the jalapeño. Serve topped with the cilantro.

Make-ahead tip: Make this the day before you plan to eat it and store refrigerated in a covered container. The flavors will mingle during storage and taste even better the next day.

Complete the Plate: Add a hearty soup or salad that contains both veggies and nourishing quality carbohydrates. I recommend carrying the curry flavor throughout the meal with Curried Carrot Soup (page 94), or try Tomato and Kale Soup (page 91).

PER SERVING: Calories: 140; Total Fat: 7g; Protein: 18g; Carbohydrates: 3g; Sugars: 1g; Fiber: 1g; Sodium: 141mg

Asian-Style Grilled Beef Salad

Gluten-Free | Dairy-Free | Nut-Free | 30 Minutes or Less

Enjoy the sweet and savory goodness of grilled flank steak on a bed of fresh summer vegetables in this Asian-inspired salad. Slice the steak thinly and enjoy a low-carb, nutrient-dense meal that will satisfy all of your taste buds.

CARBS PER SERVING: 10g
SERVINGS: 4
PREP TIME: 15 minutes
COOK TIME: 15 minutes

FOR THE DRESSING

¼ cup freshly squeezed lime juice

1 tablespoon low-sodium tamari or gluten-free soy sauce

1 tablespoon extra-virgin olive oil

1 garlic clove, minced

1 teaspoon honey

¼ teaspoon red pepper flakes

FOR THE SALAD

1 pound grass-fed flank steak

¼ teaspoon salt

Pinch freshly ground black pepper

6 cups chopped leaf lettuce

1 cucumber, halved lengthwise and thinly cut into half moons

½ small red onion, sliced

1 carrot, cut into ribbons

¼ cup chopped fresh cilantro

TO MAKE THE DRESSING

In a small bowl, whisk together the lime juice, tamari, olive oil, garlic, honey, and red pepper flakes. Set aside.

TO MAKE THE SALAD

1. Season the beef on both sides with the salt and pepper.

2. Heat a skillet over high heat until hot. Cook the beef for 3 to 6 minutes per side, depending on preferred doneness. Set aside, tented with aluminum foil, for 10 minutes.

3. In a large bowl, toss the lettuce, cucumber, onion, carrot, and cilantro.

4. Slice the beef thinly against the grain and transfer to the salad bowl.

5. Drizzle with the dressing and toss. Serve.

Substitution tip: To save on prep time, use a packaged, prewashed baby greens salad mix in place of the chopped lettuce.

Complete the Plate: Serve with a few slices of avocado to add some satisfying healthy fat and a cup of your favorite berries to provide additional high-fiber, antioxidant-rich carbohydrates.

PER SERVING: Calories: 231; Total Fat: 10g; Protein: 26g; Carbohydrates: 10g; Sugars: 4g; Fiber: 2g; Sodium: 349mg

Mustard-Glazed Pork Chops

Gluten-Free | Dairy-Free | Nut-Free | 5-Ingredient | 30 Minutes or Less

These easy glazed pork chops require only four ingredients to really make them stand out. They are juicy, tender, and subtly sweet. Roast your favorite vegetables alongside them to create a simple one-pan meal.

CARBS PER SERVING: 7g
SERVINGS: 4
PREP TIME: 5 minutes
COOK TIME: 25 minutes

¼ cup Dijon mustard

1 tablespoon pure maple syrup

2 tablespoons rice vinegar

4 bone-in, thin-cut pork chops

1. Preheat the oven to 400°F.

2. In a small saucepan, combine the mustard, maple syrup, and rice vinegar. Stir to mix and bring to a simmer over medium heat. Cook for about 2 minutes until just slightly thickened.

3. In a baking dish, place the pork chops and spoon the sauce over them, flipping to coat.

4. Bake, uncovered, for 18 to 22 minutes until the juices run clear.

Substitution tip: Use about 2 teaspoons of honey in place of the maple syrup.

Complete the Plate: Add at least 2 cups of roasted vegetables and up to ⅔ cup of your favorite starch to complete the plate.

PER SERVING: Calories: 257; Total Fat: 7g; Protein: 39g; Carbohydrates: 7g; Sugars: 4g; Fiber: 0g; Sodium: 466mg

Parmesan-Crusted Pork Chops

Gluten-Free | Nut-Free | 5-Ingredient

These quick and crispy baked pork chops are deliciously simple to make and yet another great option for an easy weeknight meal. I love the addition of Parmesan cheese, since it is a natural cheese that has bold flavor, yet portions can be kept small without sacrificing any of the taste. I love to eat this with roasted vegetables, which can be baked at the same time as the pork chops to save time and energy in the kitchen. This Parmesan topping also works well on white fish, such as tilapia or mahi mahi, as well as poultry.

CARBS PER SERVING: 1g

SERVINGS: 4

PREP TIME: 10 minutes

COOK TIME: 25 minutes

Nonstick cooking spray

4 bone-in, thin-cut pork chops

2 tablespoons butter

½ cup grated Parmesan cheese

3 garlic cloves, minced

¼ teaspoon salt

¼ teaspoon dried thyme

Freshly ground black pepper

1. Preheat the oven to 400°F. Line a baking sheet with parchment paper and spray with nonstick cooking spray.

2. Arrange the pork chops on the prepared baking sheet so they do not overlap.

3. In a small bowl, combine the butter, cheese, garlic, salt, thyme, and pepper. Press 2 tablespoons of the cheese mixture onto the top of each pork chop.

4. Bake for 18 to 22 minutes until the pork is cooked through and its juices run clear. Set the broiler to high, then broil for 1 to 2 minutes to brown the tops.

Ingredient tip: **Look for butter made from grass-fed cows, which provides higher amounts of vitamin A and omega-3 fatty acids.**

Complete the Plate: Pair with at least 2 cups of nonstarchy vegetables and a starchy side dish. Examples include Green Salad with Blackberries, Goat Cheese, and Sweet Potatoes (page 103) or Comforting Summer Squash Soup with Crispy Chickpeas (page 92).

PER SERVING: Calories: 332; Total Fat: 16g; Protein: 44g; Carbohydrates: 1g; Sugars: 0g; Fiber: 0g; Sodium: 440mg

Mango-Glazed Pork Tenderloin Roast

Gluten-Free | Dairy-Free | Nut-Free | 30 Minutes or Less

Fresh parsley and rosemary create an irresistible flavor combo with this roasted pork tenderloin. This dish also looks beautiful, with the bright yellow-and-green color combination from the mango and herbs. With the amazing aromas that waft through your kitchen as you roast this dish, you will hardly be able to wait to sit down to your meal.

CARBS PER SERVING: 12g

SERVINGS: 4

PREP TIME: 10 minutes

COOK TIME: 20 minutes

1 pound boneless pork tenderloin, trimmed of fat

1 teaspoon chopped fresh rosemary

1 teaspoon chopped fresh thyme

¼ teaspoon salt, divided

¼ teaspoon freshly ground black pepper, divided

1 teaspoon extra-virgin olive oil

1 tablespoon honey

2 tablespoons white wine vinegar

2 tablespoons dry cooking wine

1 tablespoon minced fresh ginger

1 cup diced mango

1. Preheat the oven to 400°F.

2. Season the tenderloin with the rosemary, thyme, ⅛ teaspoon of salt, and ⅛ teaspoon of pepper.

3. Heat the olive oil in an oven-safe skillet over medium-high heat, and sear the tenderloin until browned on all sides, about 5 minutes total.

4. Transfer the skillet to the oven and roast for 12 to 15 minutes until the pork is cooked through, the juices run clear, and the internal temperature reaches 145°F. Transfer to a cutting board to rest for 5 minutes.

5. In a small bowl, combine the honey, vinegar, cooking wine, and ginger. In to the same skillet, pour the honey mixture and simmer for 1 minute. Add the mango and toss to coat. Transfer to a blender and purée until smooth. Season with the remaining ⅛ teaspoon of salt and ⅛ teaspoon of pepper.

6. Slice the pork into rounds and serve with the mango sauce.

●➤

Mango-Glazed Pork Tenderloin Roast, *continued*

Make-ahead tip: **Prepare the mango sauce, and measure the spices and rub the pork with them the night before, and all you have to do is toss the tenderloin in the oven when you are ready to cook.**

 Complete the Plate: **Create an easy, complete meal by adding ½ cup of your favorite starchy vegetables (green peas, winter squash, sweet potatoes, etc.) and 1 to 2 cups of nonstarchy vegetables of your choice.**

PER SERVING: Calories: 182; Total Fat: 4g; Protein: 24g; Carbohydrates: 12g; Sugars: 10g; Fiber: 1g; Sodium: 240mg

Curried Pork and Vegetable Kebabs

Gluten-Free | Nut-Free

Pork tenderloin is a versatile lean protein that takes on the powerful flavors of the herbs and spices in this dish. Turmeric has been found to fight inflammation, improve the immune system response, increase antibodies, and act as an antibacterial agent in the body. Turmeric is also best absorbed by your body to obtain these amazing benefits when it is paired with black pepper, so the combo of both in this dish is very strategic.

CARBS PER SERVING: 10g

SERVINGS: 4

PREP TIME: 15 minutes, plus 1 hour to marinate

COOK TIME: 15 minutes

¼ cup plain nonfat Greek yogurt

2 tablespoons curry powder

1 teaspoon garlic powder

1 teaspoon ground turmeric

Zest and juice of 1 lime

¼ teaspoon salt

Pinch freshly ground black pepper

1 pound boneless pork tenderloin, cut into bite-size pieces

1 red bell pepper, seeded and cut into 2-inch squares

1 green bell pepper, seeded and cut into 2-inch squares

1 red onion, quartered and split into segments

1. In a large bowl, mix the yogurt, curry powder, garlic powder, turmeric, lime zest, lime juice, salt, and pepper.

2. Add the pieces of pork tenderloin to the bowl, and stir to coat. Refrigerate for at least 1 hour or as long as 6 hours.

3. Preheat a grill or broiler to medium.

4. Thread the pork pieces, bell peppers, and onions onto skewers.

5. Grill or broil for 12 to 15 minutes, flipping every 3 or 4 minutes, until the pork is cooked through. Serve.

Technique tip: If you're using wooden skewers, be sure to soak them for at least 30 minutes before threading the meat and vegetables on them to prevent scorching during cooking.

 Complete the Plate: Serve with an additional 1 to 2 servings of carbohydrates as well as another healthy fat source. A simple addition would be ½ cup quinoa topped with a few slices of avocado.

PER SERVING: Calories: 175; Total Fat: 3g; Protein: 27g; Carbohydrates: 10g; Sugars: 4g; Fiber: 3g; Sodium: 188mg

Lamb, Mushroom, and Goat Cheese Burgers

Gluten-Free | Nut-Free | 5-Ingredient | 30 Minutes or Less

Get ready to take your grilling skills to the next level with these gourmet lamb burgers! The mushrooms add an extra savory flavor to the burgers, while the blend of goat cheese and basil provides an impressive and unexpected flavor combo. Don't be surprised if all your guests ask for seconds at your next barbecue!

CARBS PER SERVING: 3g

SERVINGS: 4

PREP TIME: 15 minutes

COOK TIME: 15 minutes

8 ounces grass-fed ground lamb

8 ounces brown mushrooms, finely chopped

¼ teaspoon salt

¼ teaspoon freshly ground black pepper

¼ cup crumbled goat cheese

1 tablespoon minced fresh basil

1. In a large mixing bowl, combine the lamb, mushrooms, salt, and pepper, and mix well.

2. In a small bowl, mix the goat cheese and basil.

3. Form the lamb mixture into 4 patties, reserving about ½ cup of the mixture in the bowl. In each patty, make an indentation in the center and fill with 1 tablespoon of the goat cheese mixture. Use the reserved meat mixture to close the burgers. Press the meat firmly to hold together.

4. Heat the barbecue or a large skillet over medium-high heat. Add the burgers and cook for 5 to 7 minutes on each side, until cooked through. Serve.

Substitution tip: If you don't like the tang of goat cheese, substitute feta.

 Complete the Plate: Serve on a whole-wheat bun or with classic sweet potato oven fries, along with Cabbage Slaw Salad (page 102) or a simple green salad with Ranch Vegetable Dip and Dressing (page 239).

PER SERVING: Calories: 173; Total Fat: 13g; Protein: 11g; Carbohydrates: 3g; Sugars: 1g; Fiber: 0g; Sodium: 154mg

Lamb Chops with Cherry Glaze

Gluten-Free | Dairy-Free | Nut-Free | 30 Minutes or Less

Cherry season lasts only about three months in the United States, but with the help of frozen cherries, the powerful antioxidants found in them are available year-round. This simple and healthy glaze is the perfect complement to these seared lamb chops and is delicious enough to turn any occasion into a celebration.

CARBS PER SERVING: 6g

SERVINGS: 4

PREP TIME: 10 minutes

COOK TIME: 20 minutes

4 (4-ounce) lamb chops

1½ teaspoons chopped fresh rosemary

¼ teaspoon salt

¼ teaspoon freshly ground black pepper

1 cup frozen cherries, thawed

¼ cup dry red wine

2 tablespoons orange juice

1 teaspoon extra-virgin olive oil

1. Season the lamb chops with the rosemary, salt, and pepper.

2. In a small saucepan over medium-low heat, combine the cherries, red wine, and orange juice, and simmer, stirring regularly, until the sauce thickens, 8 to 10 minutes.

3. Heat a large skillet over medium-high heat. When the pan is hot, add the olive oil to lightly coat the bottom.

4. Cook the lamb chops for 3 to 4 minutes on each side until well-browned yet medium rare.

5. Serve, topped with the cherry glaze.

Make-ahead tip: Make the cherry glaze up to 2 days in advance and store in the refrigerator until you're ready to use it.

Complete the Plate: Add 1 to 2 servings of carbohydrates in the form of fruit or a starch, such as Three Bean and Basil Salad (page 105), along with at least 2 cups of your favorite nonstarchy vegetables.

PER SERVING: Calories: 356; Total Fat: 27g; Protein: 20g; Carbohydrates: 6g; Sugars: 4g; Fiber: 1g; Sodium: 199mg

Slow-Cooked Simple Lamb and Vegetable Stew

Gluten-Free | Dairy-Free | Nut-Free | Slow Cooker Easy

I wish I could personally thank the creator of the slow cooker, because it is without a doubt my favorite appliance in my kitchen. Throwing everything into one pot and coming back to a delicious meal a few hours later is nothing short of magical to me. I hope this stew provides the warm nourishment you are looking for during the cool winter months.

CARBS PER SERVING: 27g
SERVINGS: 6
PREP TIME: 10 minutes
COOK TIME: 3 to 6 hours

1 pound boneless lamb stew meat

1 pound turnips, peeled and chopped

1 fennel bulb, trimmed and thinly sliced

10 ounces mushrooms, sliced

1 onion, diced

3 garlic cloves, minced

2 cups low-sodium chicken broth

2 tablespoons tomato paste

¼ cup dry red wine (optional)

1 teaspoon chopped fresh thyme

½ teaspoon salt

¼ teaspoon freshly ground black pepper

Chopped fresh parsley, for garnish

1. In a slow cooker, combine the lamb, turnips, fennel, mushrooms, onion, garlic, chicken broth, tomato paste, red wine (if using), thyme, salt, and pepper.

2. Cover and cook on high for 3 hours or on low for 6 hours. When the meat is tender and falling apart, garnish with parsley and serve.

3. If you don't have a slow cooker, in a large pot, heat 2 teaspoons of olive oil over medium heat, and sear the lamb on all sides. Remove from the pot and set aside. Add the turnips, fennel, mushrooms, onion, and garlic to the pot, and cook for 3 to 4 minutes until the vegetables begin to soften. Add the chicken broth, tomato paste, red wine (if using), thyme, salt, pepper, and browned lamb. Bring to a boil, then reduce the heat to low. Simmer for 1½ to 2 hours until the meat is tender. Garnish with parsley and serve.

Option tip: For a spicy stew, add a seeded and minced jalapeño pepper.

 Complete the Plate: This is a well-balanced plate, so enjoy as is. Or you can add another serving of vegetables and/or carbohydrates.

PER SERVING: Calories: 303; Total Fat: 7g; Protein: 32g; Carbohydrates: 27g; Sugars: 7g; Fiber: 4g; Sodium: 310mg

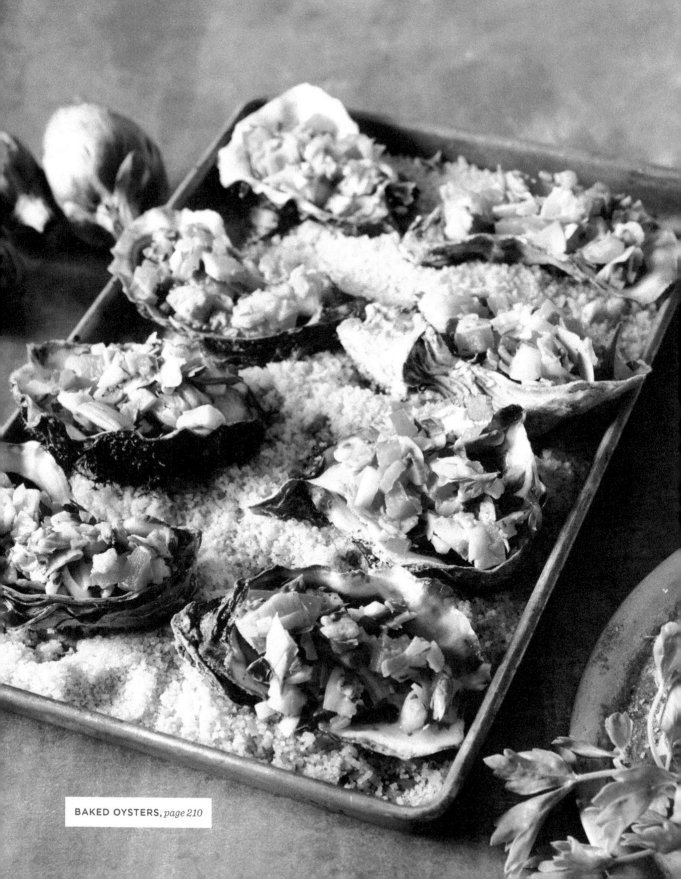

BAKED OYSTERS, *page 210*

12

Fish and Seafood

Tomato Tuna Melts

Gluten-Free | Nut-Free | 30 Minutes or Less

With the help of these Tomato Tuna Melts, you'll never have to suffer through a bland or boring lunch again. They are one of my go-to lunch favorites, because they're ready in minutes and give me the energy to power through the rest of my day. And without the bread, they're way lower in carbs than the old-school cafeteria version.

CARBS PER SERVING: 7g
SERVINGS: 2
PREP TIME: 5 minutes
COOK TIME: 5 minutes

1 (5-ounce) can chunk light tuna packed in water, drained

2 tablespoons plain nonfat Greek yogurt

2 teaspoons freshly squeezed lemon juice

2 tablespoons finely chopped celery

1 tablespoon finely chopped red onion

Pinch cayenne pepper

1 large tomato, cut into ¾-inch-thick rounds

½ cup shredded cheddar cheese

1. Preheat the broiler to high.

2. In a medium bowl, combine the tuna, yogurt, lemon juice, celery, red onion, and cayenne pepper. Stir well.

3. Arrange the tomato slices on a baking sheet. Top each with some tuna salad and cheddar cheese.

4. Broil for 3 to 4 minutes until the cheese is melted and bubbly. Serve.

Make-ahead tip: You can make the tuna salad up to 3 days in advance. Cover and refrigerate single servings so the melts are ready to assemble, broil, and serve. If you have access to a microwave at work, you can assemble the melts and then finish them in the microwave in about 20 to 30 seconds.

 Complete the Plate: It's a good idea to add an additional serving of vegetables and carbohydrates to this meal to add enough fiber and create a filling, balanced meal. I recommend Mushroom and Pesto Flatbread Pizza (page 134); Brussels Sprout, Avocado, and Wild Rice Bowl (page 137); or simply some whole-grain crackers with a side salad.

PER SERVING: Calories: 243; Total Fat: 10g; Protein: 30g; Carbohydrates: 7g; Sugars: 2g; Fiber: 1g; Sodium: 444mg

Peppercorn-Crusted Baked Salmon

Gluten-Free | Dairy-Free | Nut-Free | 5-Ingredient | 30 Minutes or Less

Simple meals will always be the best to me, because they can realistically be included in your weekly eating plans for weeks and years to come—and that's exactly what we all need in order to make long-term changes. I hope this baked salmon will remind you that you always have the option to choose healthy and accessible foods, as long as you are willing to commit 30 minutes (or less!) to prepare it.

CARBS PER SERVING: 1g
SERVINGS: 4
PREP TIME: 5 minutes
COOK TIME: 20 minutes

Nonstick cooking spray

½ teaspoon freshly ground black pepper

¼ teaspoon salt

Zest and juice of ½ lemon

¼ teaspoon dried thyme

1 pound salmon fillet

1. Preheat the oven to 425°F. Spray a baking sheet with nonstick cooking spray.

2. In a small bowl, combine the pepper, salt, lemon zest and juice, and thyme. Stir to combine.

3. Place the salmon on the prepared baking sheet, skin-side down. Spread the seasoning mixture evenly over the fillet.

4. Bake for 15 to 20 minutes, depending on the thickness of the fillet, until the flesh flakes easily.

Option tip: Add a pound of cut-up asparagus, broccoli, or cauliflower tossed with 1 teaspoon of olive oil to the baking sheet before baking to make it a meal.

Complete the Plate: Add additional servings of carbohydrates and vegetables. Keep it simple and include a small baked sweet potato and 1 or 2 cups of steamed broccoli or a green salad.

PER SERVING: Calories: 163; Total Fat: 7g; Protein: 23g; Carbohydrates: 1g; Sugars: 0g; Fiber: 0g; Sodium: 167mg

Roasted Salmon with Honey-Mustard Sauce

Gluten-Free | Dairy-Free | Nut-Free | 5-Ingredient | 30 Minutes or Less

Even if you have made salmon a thousand times, you'll still love this simple recipe. It's subtly sweet and full of flavor. You'll find this roasting in my house at least once a week. It's the easiest salmon recipe I've ever made, and I go back to it time and time again. I hope it becomes a weekly go-to that finds its way into your home, as well.

CARBS PER SERVING: 6g
SERVINGS: 4
PREP TIME: 5 minutes
COOK TIME: 20 minutes

Nonstick cooking spray

2 tablespoons whole-grain mustard

1 tablespoon honey

2 garlic cloves, minced

¼ teaspoon salt

¼ teaspoon freshly ground black pepper

1 pound salmon fillet

1. Preheat the oven to 425°F. Spray a baking sheet with non-stick cooking spray.

2. In a small bowl, whisk together the mustard, honey, garlic, salt, and pepper.

3. Place the salmon fillet on the prepared baking sheet, skin-side down. Spoon the sauce onto the salmon and spread evenly.

4. Roast for 15 to 20 minutes, depending on the thickness of the fillet, until the flesh flakes easily.

Substitution tip: If you don't have whole-grain mustard, Dijon will be just fine.

 Complete the Plate: Serve with an additional serving of vegetables and carbohydrates. An easy addition is Warm Barley and Squash Salad with Balsamic Vinaigrette (page 107).

PER SERVING: Calories: 186; Total Fat: 7g; Protein: 23g; Carbohydrates: 6g; Sugars: 4g; Fiber: 0g; Sodium: 312mg

Ginger-Glazed Salmon and Broccoli

Gluten-Free   Dairy-Free   Nut-Free   30 Minutes or Less

Ginger is one of the healthiest spices in the world. Over the years, research has found it to lower inflammation, improve digestion, improve brain function, and even prevent cancer. But most importantly for people newly diagnosed with diabetes, a 2015 study found it lowered fasting blood sugar levels and overall hemoglobin A1c levels. So in case you needed another reason to enjoy ginger regularly, there you go!

CARBS PER SERVING: 11g

SERVINGS: 4

PREP TIME: 10 minutes

COOK TIME: 15 minutes

Nonstick cooking spray

1 tablespoon low-sodium tamari or gluten-free soy sauce

Juice of 1 lemon

1 tablespoon honey

1 (1-inch) piece fresh ginger, grated

1 garlic clove, minced

1 pound salmon fillet

¼ teaspoon salt, divided

⅛ teaspoon freshly ground black pepper

2 broccoli heads, cut into florets

1 tablespoon extra-virgin olive oil

1. Preheat the oven to 400°F. Spray a baking sheet with non-stick cooking spray.

2. In a small bowl, mix the tamari, lemon juice, honey, ginger, and garlic. Set aside.

3. Place the salmon skin-side down on the prepared baking sheet. Season with ⅛ teaspoon of salt and the pepper.

4. In a large mixing bowl, toss the broccoli and olive oil. Season with the remaining ⅛ teaspoon of salt. Arrange in a single layer on the baking sheet next to the salmon. Bake for 15 to 20 minutes until the salmon flakes easily with a fork and the broccoli is fork-tender.

◆➤

5. In a small pan over medium heat, bring the tamari-ginger mixture to a simmer and cook for 1 to 2 minutes until it just begins to thicken.

6. Drizzle the sauce over the salmon and serve.

Substitution tip: Asparagus works well in place of the broccoli. Use 1 pound of asparagus, trimmed, and cook the same as instructed in steps 4 and 5.

 Complete the Plate: If desired, add another serving of vegetables and carbohydrates. I enjoy Roasted Delicata Squash (page 125) and/or Three Bean and Basil Salad (page 105) with this dish.

PER SERVING: Calories: 238; Total Fat: 11g; Protein: 25g; Carbohydrates: 11g; Sugars: 6g; Fiber: 2g; Sodium: 334mg

Roasted Salmon with Salsa Verde

Gluten-Free | Dairy-Free | Nut-Free | 30 Minutes or Less

A simple, well-cooked piece of salmon is the highlight of this meal. You probably don't need me to remind you of the many benefits of salmon, but it is frequently referred to as a superfood, and for good reason. What you may not know is that the omega-3 fats in salmon have been found to prevent heart disease, lower blood pressure, and relieve symptoms of depression. If you're really in a hurry with this dish, you can buy store-bought salsa verde instead of making your own.

CARBS PER SERVING: 6g

SERVINGS: 4

PREP TIME: 5 minutes

COOK TIME: 25 minutes

Nonstick cooking spray

8 ounces tomatillos, husks removed

½ onion, quartered

1 jalapeño or serrano pepper, seeded

1 garlic clove, unpeeled

1 teaspoon extra-virgin olive oil

½ teaspoon salt, divided

4 (4-ounce) wild-caught salmon fillets

¼ teaspoon freshly ground black pepper

¼ cup chopped fresh cilantro

Juice of 1 lime

1. Preheat the oven to 425°F. Spray a baking sheet with non-stick cooking spray.

2. In a large bowl, toss the tomatillos, onion, jalapeño, garlic, olive oil, and ¼ teaspoon of salt to coat. Arrange in a single layer on the prepared baking sheet, and roast for about 10 minutes until just softened. Transfer to a dish or plate and set aside.

3. Arrange the salmon fillets skin-side down on the same baking sheet, and season with the remaining ¼ teaspoon of salt and the pepper. Bake for 12 to 15 minutes until the fish is firm and flakes easily.

➡

4. Meanwhile, peel the roasted garlic and place it and the roasted vegetables in a blender or food processor. Add a scant ¼ cup of water to the jar, and process until smooth.

5. Add the cilantro and lime juice and process until smooth. Serve the salmon topped with the salsa verde.

Ingredient tip: Tomatillos are also known as husk or Mexican tomatoes and are a staple in Mexican cuisine. They can be can be eaten raw or cooked, after you remove the papery husk and rinse them. You can probably find them in your local grocery store, but if not, you can definitely find them in a Latino grocery.

Complete the Plate: **Complete this Mexican-inspired meal with Cucumber, Tomato, Avocado Salad (page 101) and Rainbow Black Bean Salad (page 106).**

PER SERVING: Calories: 199; Total Fat: 9g; Protein: 23g; Carbohydrates: 6g; Sugars: 3g; Fiber: 2g; Sodium: 295mg

Ceviche

Gluten-Free | Dairy-Free | Nut-Free | No-Cook

Ceviche is a popular dish made of raw fish marinated (almost "cooked") in citrus juices. Most people don't prepare it at home, but it is surprisingly easy (and delicious!). Make it as spicy as you like, and keep it low carb by skipping the tostadas and serving it instead with a filling bean salad or simple boiled black beans to make it a complete meal.

CARBS PER SERVING: 11g

SERVINGS: 4

PREP TIME: 10 minutes, plus 4 hours to marinate

½ pound fresh skinless, white, ocean fish fillet (halibut, mahi mahi, etc.), diced

1 cup freshly squeezed lime juice, divided

2 tablespoons chopped fresh cilantro, divided

1 serrano pepper, sliced

1 garlic clove, crushed

¾ teaspoon salt, divided

½ red onion, thinly sliced

2 tomatoes, diced

1 red bell pepper, seeded and diced

1 tablespoon extra-virgin olive oil

1. In a large mixing bowl, combine the fish, ¾ cup of lime juice, 1 tablespoon of cilantro, serrano pepper, garlic, and ½ teaspoon of salt. The fish should be covered or nearly covered in lime juice. Cover the bowl and refrigerate for 4 hours.

2. Sprinkle the remaining ¼ teaspoon of salt over the onion in a small bowl, and let sit for 10 minutes. Drain and rinse well.

3. In a large bowl, combine the tomatoes, bell pepper, olive oil, remaining ¼ cup of lime juice, and onion. Let rest for at least 10 minutes, or as long as 4 hours, while the fish "cooks."

4. When the fish is ready, it will be completely white and opaque. At this time, strain the juice, reserving it in another bowl. If desired, remove the serrano pepper and garlic.

➤

5. Add the vegetables to the fish, and stir gently. Taste, and add some of the reserved lime juice to the ceviche as desired. Serve topped with the remaining 1 tablespoon of cilantro.

Make-ahead tip: Ceviche can be made up to 1 day in advance. However, if you are making it more than 4 hours ahead, be sure to drain the juice so the fish does not become too tangy. Also, wait to add the vegetables until right before serving for the best flavor.

Complete the Plate: Serve with ½ cup of your favorite beans or Rainbow Black Bean Salad (page 106) along with Cucumber, Tomato, Avocado Salad (page 101).

PER SERVING: Calories: 121; Total Fat: 4g; Protein: 12g; Carbohydrates: 11g; Sugars: 5g; Fiber: 2g; Sodium: 405mg

Whole Veggie-Stuffed Trout

Gluten-Free | Dairy-Free | Nut-Free

If you aren't already a huge fan of trout, I hope this dish will convince you. Trout is rich in a specific type of omega-3 fat, called DHA, that is essential for brain health. In fact, eating adequate levels of DHA throughout your life has been associated with improved memory and reduced levels of cognitive decline.

CARBS PER SERVING: 14g
SERVINGS: 2
PREP TIME: 10 minutes
COOK TIME: 25 minutes

Nonstick cooking spray

2 (8-ounce) whole trout fillets, dressed (cleaned but with bones and skin intact)

1 tablespoon extra-virgin olive oil

¼ teaspoon salt

⅛ teaspoon freshly ground black pepper

½ red bell pepper, seeded and thinly sliced

1 small onion, thinly sliced

2 or 3 shiitake mushrooms, sliced

1 poblano pepper, seeded and thinly sliced

1 lemon, sliced

1. Preheat the oven to 425°F. Spray a baking sheet with non-stick cooking spray.

2. Rub both trout, inside and out, with the olive oil, then season with the salt and pepper.

3. In a large bowl, combine the bell pepper, onion, mushrooms, and poblano pepper. Stuff half of this mixture into the cavity of each fish. Top the mixture with 2 or 3 lemon slices inside each fish.

4. Arrange the fish on the prepared baking sheet side by side and roast for 25 minutes until the fish is cooked through and the vegetables are tender.

Make-ahead tip: Stuff the fish the night before, wrap in plastic wrap, and refrigerate, and you'll have this ready to go into the oven when you walk in the door after a long day.

Complete the Plate: This is a very satisfying dish by itself, but if you are looking to add another serving of carbs, consider adding ½ cup of your favorite berries or ½ cup of a starch or whole grain.

PER SERVING: Calories: 452; Total Fat: 22g; Protein: 49g; Carbohydrates: 14g; Sugars: 5g; Fiber: 3g; Sodium: 357mg

Ginger-Garlic Cod Cooked in Paper

Gluten-Free | Dairy-Free | Nut-Free | 30 Minutes or Less

I always make sure to have a bag of frozen cod in my freezer, since it is one of the most versatile types of fish, is quick to cook, and offers plenty of health benefits. Cod is also very lean, with only 1 gram of fat per 3-ounce portion. Since most major health organizations encourage eating fish at least twice per week, I hope this recipe gives you a good reason to go with cod. Enjoy!

CARBS PER SERVING: 9g

SERVINGS: 4

PREP TIME: 10 minutes

COOK TIME: 15 minutes

1 chard bunch, stemmed, leaves and stems cut into thin strips

1 red bell pepper, seeded and cut into strips

1 pound cod fillets cut into 4 pieces

1 tablespoon grated fresh ginger

3 garlic cloves, minced

2 tablespoons white wine vinegar

2 tablespoons low-sodium tamari or gluten-free soy sauce

1 tablespoon honey

1. Preheat the oven to 425°F.

2. Cut four pieces of parchment paper, each about 16 inches wide. Lay the four pieces out on a large workspace.

3. On each piece of paper, arrange a small pile of chard leaves and stems, topped by several strips of bell pepper. Top with a piece of cod.

4. In a small bowl, mix the ginger, garlic, vinegar, tamari, and honey. Top each piece of fish with one-fourth of the mixture.

5. Fold the parchment paper over so the edges overlap. Fold the edges over several times to secure the fish in the packets. Carefully place the packets on a large baking sheet.

6. Bake for 12 minutes. Carefully open the packets, allowing steam to escape, and serve.

Substitution tip: Bok choy, zucchini, and other quick-cooking vegetables work well when cooked this way. Experiment with your favorites to find your own unique combination.

 Complete the Plate: While this provides a good amount of lean protein and veggies, you will definitely want to add more healthy fat and carbohydrates to create a balanced plate. I think this dish tastes great with Three Bean and Basil Salad (page 105) and Green Bean Casserole (page 127).

PER SERVING: Calories: 118; Total Fat: 1g; Protein: 19g; Carbohydrates: 9g; Sugars: 6g; Fiber: 1g; Sodium: 715mg

Roasted Halibut with Red Peppers, Green Beans, and Onions

Gluten-Free | Dairy-Free | Nut-Free | 30 Minutes or Less

Halibut is an amazing addition to any meal. It is generally less expensive than other types of fish, yet the nutritional benefits are profound. Halibut contains brain-boosting omega-3 fatty acids, magnesium, potassium, B vitamins, and blood sugar–stabilizing protein.

CARBS PER SERVING: 16g

SERVINGS: 4

PREP TIME: 10 minutes

COOK TIME: 15 minutes

1 pound green beans, trimmed

2 red bell peppers, seeded and cut into strips

1 onion, sliced

Zest and juice of 2 lemons

3 garlic cloves, minced

2 tablespoons extra-virgin olive oil

1 teaspoon dried dill

1 teaspoon dried oregano

4 (4-ounce) halibut fillets

½ teaspoon salt

¼ teaspoon freshly ground black pepper

1. Preheat the oven to 400°F. Line a baking sheet with parchment paper.

2. In a large bowl, toss the green beans, bell peppers, onion, lemon zest and juice, garlic, olive oil, dill, and oregano.

3. Use a slotted spoon to transfer the vegetables to the prepared baking sheet in a single layer, leaving the juice behind in the bowl.

4. Gently place the halibut fillets in the bowl, and coat in the juice. Transfer the fillets to the baking sheet, nestled between the vegetables, and drizzle them with any juice left in the bowl. Sprinkle the vegetables and halibut with the salt and pepper.

5. Bake for 15 to 20 minutes until the vegetables are just tender and the fish flakes apart easily.

Technique tip: Using parchment paper makes cleanup easy, especially when roasting, as the fish oils can get burned on to baking sheets and be hard to remove. This technique is cost-effective and saves you time, making parchment paper a great kitchen tool you should use regularly.

 Complete the Plate: While this recipe contains all the elements of a complete meal, you may want to add more carbohydrates and healthy fat to ensure you are full and energized. I enjoy combining this dish with Rainbow Black Bean Salad (page 106) or Three Bean and Basil Salad (page 105).

PER SERVING: Calories: 234; Total Fat: 9g; Protein: 24g; Carbohydrates: 16g; Sugars: 8g; Fiber: 5g; Sodium: 349mg

Blackened Tilapia with Mango Salsa

Gluten-Free | Dairy-Free | Nut-Free | 30 Minutes or Less

Tilapia has a mild and delicate flavor and often turns up in the freezer section at the supermarket. Fresh mango salsa definitely adds unique, tropical flavor to this dish. In fact, this salsa is a perfect addition to any grilled fish or favorite lean protein, especially at the end of a long summer day. I hope you enjoy it often, and feel free to change the recipe as desired to make it your own.

CARBS PER SERVING: 22g

SERVINGS: 2

PREP TIME: 15 minutes

COOK TIME: 10 minutes

FOR THE SALSA

1 cup chopped mango

2 tablespoons chopped red onion

2 tablespoons chopped fresh cilantro

2 tablespoons freshly squeezed lime juice

½ jalapeño pepper, seeded and minced

Pinch salt

TO MAKE THE SALSA

In a medium bowl, toss together the mango, onion, cilantro, lime juice, jalapeño, and salt. Set aside.

FOR THE TILAPIA

1 tablespoon paprika

1 teaspoon onion powder

½ teaspoon freshly ground black pepper

½ teaspoon dried thyme

½ teaspoon garlic powder

¼ teaspoon cayenne pepper

¼ teaspoon salt

½ pound boneless tilapia fillets

2 teaspoons extra-virgin olive oil

1 lime, cut into wedges, for serving

TO MAKE THE TILAPIA

1. In a small bowl, mix the paprika, onion powder, pepper, thyme, garlic powder, cayenne, and salt. Rub the mixture on both sides of the tilapia fillets.

2. In a large skillet, heat the oil over medium heat, and cook the fish for 3 to 5 minutes on each side until the outer coating is crisp and the fish is cooked through.

3. Spoon half of the salsa over each fillet and serve with lime wedges on the side.

Substitution tip: Pineapple salsa also pairs well with the heat of this dish. Substitute an equal amount of fresh or canned pineapple for the mango.

 Complete the Plate: Add your favorite nonstarchy vegetables, like Cucumber, Tomato, and Avocado Salad (page 101) or Roasted Asparagus, Onions, and Red Peppers (page 126).

PER SERVING: Calories: 240; Total Fat: 8g; Protein: 25g; Carbohydrates: 22g; Sugars: 13g; Fiber: 4g; Sodium: 417mg

Scallops and Asparagus Skillet

Gluten-Free | Dairy-Free | Nut-Free | 30 Minutes or Less

Scallops are always my favorite choice when I am dining out at a seafood restaurant, but they are very easy to make at home, too. You can buy frozen scallops to have on hand to make this simple gourmet meal in less than half an hour any day of the week. Scallops are especially healthy because they contain a significant amount of magnesium, one of the minerals that is commonly low in people with type 2 diabetes.

CARBS PER SERVING: 15g
SERVINGS: 4
PREP TIME: 10 minutes
COOK TIME: 15 minutes

3 teaspoons extra-virgin olive oil, divided

1 pound asparagus, trimmed and cut into 2-inch segments

1 tablespoon butter

1 pound sea scallops

¼ cup dry white wine

Juice of 1 lemon

2 garlic cloves, minced

¼ teaspoon freshly ground black pepper

1. In a large skillet, heat 1½ teaspoons of oil over medium heat.

2. Add the asparagus and sauté for 5 to 6 minutes until just tender, stirring regularly. Remove from the skillet and cover with aluminum foil to keep warm.

3. Add the remaining 1½ teaspoons of oil and the butter to the skillet. When the butter is melted and sizzling, place the scallops in a single layer in the skillet. Cook for about 3 minutes on one side until nicely browned. Use tongs to gently loosen and flip the scallops, and cook on the other side for another 3 minutes until browned and cooked through. Remove and cover with foil to keep warm.

4. In the same skillet, combine the wine, lemon juice, garlic, and pepper. Bring to a simmer for 1 to 2 minutes, stirring to mix in any browned pieces left in the pan.

5. Return the asparagus and the cooked scallops to the skillet to coat with the sauce. Serve warm.

Option tip: Bok choy pairs nicely with scallops. To use, cut crosswise into thin slices and sauté with the sauce in the skillet for 5 to 6 minutes until the white parts are tender.

 Complete the Plate: While this dish satisfies all of the requirements of a full plate, I would still recommend adding an additional serving of vegetables and a healthy-carb side dish. Consider ½ cup quinoa with an additional cup of roasted vegetables to complete your quick and healthy meal.

PER SERVING: Calories: 252; Total Fat: 7g; Protein: 26g; Carbohydrates: 15g; Sugars: 3g; Fiber: 2g; Sodium: 493mg

Baked Oysters

Gluten-Free | Nut-Free

You may already know that oysters are another fantastic source of healthy omega-3 fatty acids, but they are also high in zinc, which is especially helpful for people with type 2 diabetes since zinc helps the beta cells of the pancreas create insulin. In this veggie-filled baked version, you'll find the perfect combo of fresh citrus and fragrant garlic to bring all the flavors together beautifully in a dish that will likely make oysters a more regular part of your diet.

CARBS PER SERVING: 11g

SERVINGS: 2

PREP TIME: 30 minutes

COOK TIME: 15 minutes

2 cups coarse salt, for holding the oysters

1 dozen fresh oysters, scrubbed

1 tablespoon butter

½ cup finely chopped artichoke hearts

¼ cup finely chopped scallions, both white and green parts

¼ cup finely chopped red bell pepper

1 garlic clove, minced

1 tablespoon finely chopped fresh parsley

Zest and juice of ½ lemon

Pinch salt

Freshly ground black pepper

1. Pour the coarse salt into an 8-by-8-inch baking dish and spread to evenly fill the bottom of the dish.

2. Prepare a clean surface to shuck the oysters. Using a shucking knife, insert the blade at the joint of the shell, where it hinges open and shut. Firmly apply pressure to pop the blade in, and work the knife around the shell to open. Discard the empty half of the shell. Use the knife to gently loosen the oyster, and remove any shell particles. Set the oysters in their shells on the salt, being careful not to spill the juices.

3. Preheat the oven to 425°F.

4. In a large skillet, melt the butter over medium heat. Add the artichoke hearts, scallions, and bell pepper, and cook for 5 to 7 minutes. Add the garlic and cook an additional minute. Remove from the heat and mix in the parsley, lemon zest and juice, and season with salt and pepper.

5. Divide the vegetable mixture evenly among the oysters and bake for 10 to 12 minutes until the vegetables are lightly browned.

Technique tip: An oyster-shucking knife is a necessary tool for opening oysters; don't try to shuck without one. The dull blade enables you to open the shell without cutting yourself. These knives are inexpensive and can be found at most supermarkets, often near the seafood itself.

 Complete the Plate: This dish has about 1 ounce of protein, so you will need a hearty side dish added. A great addition would be Crispy Parmesan Cups with White Beans and Veggies (page 136) and up to ½ cup cooked quinoa, if desired.

PER SERVING: Calories: 134; Total Fat: 7g; Protein: 6g; Carbohydrates: 11g; Sugars: 7g; Fiber: 2g; Sodium: 281mg

Tropical Shrimp Cocktail

Gluten-Free | Dairy-Free | Nut-Free | 30 Minutes or Less

Up your shrimp cocktail game with this tropical twist. Anyone can throw some steamed shrimp on a plate, but this version will be sure to impress. Serve it solo as an appetizer, or add it to a salad to make it a meal.

CARBS PER SERVING: 20g
SERVINGS: 4
PREP TIME: 15 minutes
COOK TIME: 3 minutes

1 pound medium shrimp, peeled and deveined

1 cup diced mango

2 ripe avocados, diced

¼ cup finely diced red onion

2 roma tomatoes, diced

¼ cup chopped fresh cilantro

2 tablespoons Low-Carb No-Cook Tomato Ketchup (page 230)

Juice of 1 lime

Juice of 1 orange

1 tablespoon extra-virgin olive oil

1 jalapeño pepper, seeded and minced

Lime wedges, for serving

1. Fill a large pot about halfway with water and bring to a boil. Meanwhile, fill a large bowl ⅔ of the way with ice and about 1 cup of cold water.

2. Add the shrimp to the boiling water and cook for 3 minutes until they are opaque and firm. Drain and quickly transfer to the ice water bath for 3 minutes to stop the cooking and cool them. Drain and pat the shrimp dry with a clean paper towel.

3. In a large bowl, mix together the shrimp, mango, avocado, red onion, tomatoes, and cilantro.

4. In a small bowl, combine the ketchup, lime juice, orange juice, oil, and jalapeño. Mix well and gently fold the sauce into the shrimp mixture.

5. Divide among 4 glasses or small dishes, with a lime wedge on the rim of each.

Make-ahead tip: To save time in the kitchen, buy precooked shrimp and start at step 3. You can also substitute a store-bought ketchup, but try to select a lower-sugar variety without high-fructose corn syrup.

 Complete the Plate: Serve with another nonstarchy vegetable and up to ½ cup of beans for a delicious and perfectly balanced Mexican-inspired meal.

PER SERVING: Calories: 279; Total Fat: 16g; Protein: 18g; Carbohydrates: 20g; Sugars: 10g; Fiber: 6g; Sodium: 676mg

Cajun Shrimp Casserole

Gluten-Free | Nut-Free

This cheesy, spicy, Louisiana-inspired casserole has just the right amount of heat from the Cajun seasoning and jalapeños, with a healthier carb option coming from the quinoa. Quinoa is a gluten-free seed (that's right, not a grain) that is considered a complete plant protein, making it a perfect substitution for white rice or pasta.

CARBS PER SERVING: 15g

SERVINGS: 6

PREP TIME: 15 minutes

COOK TIME: 30 minutes

½ cup quinoa

1 cup water

1 pound shrimp, peeled and deveined

1½ teaspoons Cajun seasoning, divided

4 tomatoes, diced

1 tablespoon plus 2 teaspoons extra-virgin olive oil, divided

½ onion, diced

1 jalapeño pepper, seeded and minced

3 garlic cloves, minced

1 tablespoon tomato paste

¼ teaspoon freshly ground black pepper

½ cup shredded pepper jack cheese

1. In a pot, combine the quinoa and water. Bring to a boil, reduce the heat, cover, and simmer on low for 10 to 15 minutes until all the water is absorbed. Fluff with a fork.

2. Preheat the oven to 350°F.

3. In a large mixing bowl, toss the shrimp and ¾ teaspoon of Cajun seasoning.

4. In another bowl, toss the remaining ¾ teaspoon of Cajun seasoning with the tomatoes and 1½ teaspoons of olive oil.

5. In a large, oven-safe skillet, heat 1 tablespoon of olive oil over medium heat. Add the shrimp and cook for 2 to 3 minutes per side until they are opaque and firm. Remove from the skillet and set aside.

6. In the same skillet, heat the remaining ½ teaspoon of olive oil over medium-high heat. Add the onion, jalapeño, and garlic, and cook until the onion softens, 3 to 5 minutes.

7. Add the seasoned tomatoes, tomato paste, cooked quinoa, and pepper. Stir well to combine.

➥

8. Return the shrimp to the skillet, placing them in a single layer on top of the quinoa. Sprinkle the cheese over the top.

9. Transfer the skillet to the oven and bake for 15 minutes. Turn the broiler on high, and broil for 2 minutes to brown the cheese. Serve.

Ingredient top: Tomato paste is usually used in small increments but is typically sold in a can, leaving you with plenty to spare. When you open a can, if you don't need to use all of it, spoon the rest into an empty ice cube tray and freeze it. Pop the cubes out, transfer to a freezer bag, and store frozen until you need them in a recipe.

 Complete the Plate: This recipe needs an additional serving of vegetables and carbs to make it complete. Consider a Brussels Sprout, Avocado, and Wild Rice Bowl (page 137) and/or Garlicky Cabbage and Collard Greens (page 121) to round out the meal.

PER SERVING: Calories: 255; Total Fat: 12g; Protein: 18g; Carbohydrates: 15g; Sugars: 1g; Fiber: 2g; Sodium: 469mg

Shrimp Burgers with Fruity Salsa and Salad

Gluten-Free | Dairy-Free | Nut-Free

If you've never made a shrimp burger, you are missing out! These flavorful, lean protein patties are easy to make and will be the perfect addition to your next outdoor barbecue. Turn up the heat by adding ½ seeded and finely chopped jalapeño pepper to the salsa. I encourage you to make a sustainable choice when it comes to the shrimp you buy, and when in doubt, check the Monterey Bay Aquarium Seafood Watch (seafoodwatch.org) list online to make the best choice you can. This is a dish that works well with frozen shrimp. Defrost them before you begin.

CARBS PER SERVING: 14g

SERVINGS: 4

PREP TIME: 15 minutes, plus 30 minutes to marinate

COOK TIME: 10 minutes

FOR THE SALSA

1 cup diced mango

1 avocado, diced

1 scallion, both white and green parts, finely chopped

1 tablespoon chopped fresh cilantro

Juice of 1 lime

¼ teaspoon freshly ground black pepper

TO MAKE THE SALSA

In a small bowl, toss the mango, avocado, scallion, and cilantro. Sprinkle with the lime juice and pepper. Mix gently to combine and set aside.

TO MAKE THE BURGERS

1. In the bowl of a food processor, add half the shrimp and process until coarsely puréed. Add the egg, bell pepper, scallions, cilantro, and garlic, and process until uniformly chopped. Transfer to a large mixing bowl.

2. Using a sharp knife, chop the remaining half pound of shrimp into small pieces. Add to the puréed mixture and stir well to combine. Add the pepper and stir well. Form the mixture into 4 patties of equal size. Arrange on a plate, cover, and refrigerate for 30 minutes.

FOR THE BURGERS

1 pound shrimp, peeled and deveined

1 large egg

½ red bell pepper, seeded and coarsely chopped

¼ cup chopped scallions, both white and green parts

2 tablespoons fresh chopped cilantro

2 garlic cloves

¼ teaspoon freshly ground black pepper

1 tablespoon extra-virgin olive oil

4 cups mixed salad greens

3. In a large skillet, heat the olive oil over medium heat. Cook the burgers for 3 minutes on each side until browned and cooked through.

4. On each of 4 plates, arrange 1 cup of salad greens, and top with a scoop of salsa and a shrimp burger.

Technique tip: If you don't have a food processor, you can use a blender to purée the shrimp. If you have neither, just chop everything really finely. The consistency won't be quite the same (the pieces will be bigger, and the burger may not hold together as well), but it should still work.

 Complete the Plate: If you prefer and your diabetes plan allows, you can serve these burgers on whole-wheat buns. Additionally, try to add another serving of your favorite vegetables. It's easy to add some roasted bell pepper to the skillet while your burger is cooking.

PER SERVING: Calories: 229; Total Fat: 11g; Protein: 19g; Carbohydrates: 14g; Sugars: 7g; Fiber: 4g; Sodium: 200mg

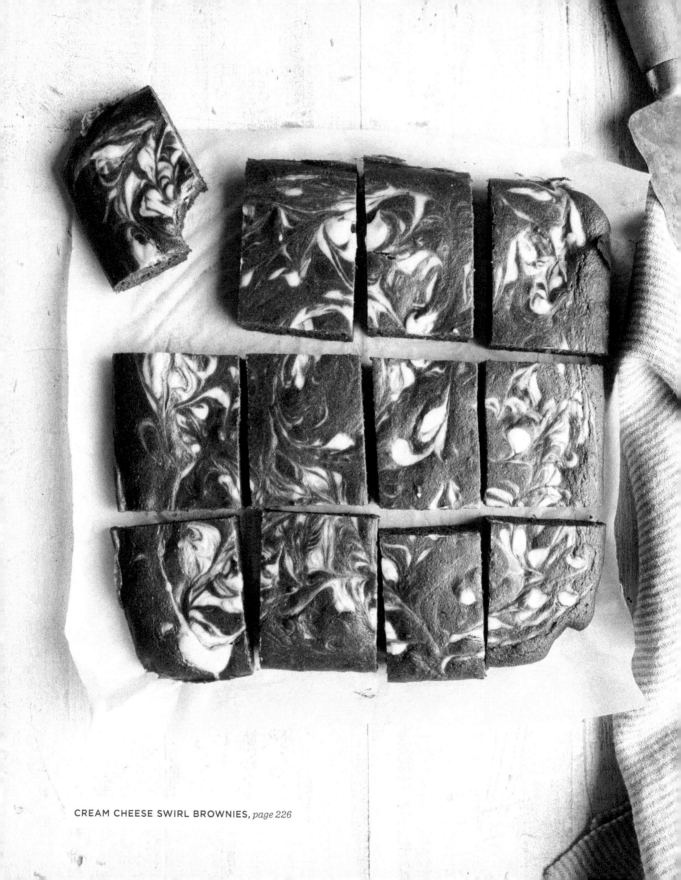

CREAM CHEESE SWIRL BROWNIES, *page 226*

13
Desserts

Berry Smoothie Pops

Gluten-Free | Vegetarian | No-Cook | 5-Ingredient | 30 Minutes or Less

Berries are at the top of my list when it comes to fruits, because they are high in fiber and antioxidants and are the fruit least likely to spike your blood sugar. These qualities make them a perfect dessert that gives you just the right amount of sweetness. Here they are combined with Greek yogurt and hemp seeds to add protein and make this dessert one that you can look forward to enjoying.

CARBS PER SERVING: 9g

SERVINGS: 6

PREP TIME: 5 minutes

2 cups frozen mixed berries

½ cup unsweetened plain almond milk

1 cup plain nonfat Greek yogurt

2 tablespoons hemp seeds

1. Place all the ingredients in a blender and process until finely blended.

2. Pour into 6 clean ice pop molds and insert sticks.

3. Freeze for 3 to 4 hours until firm.

Technique tip: Don't worry if you don't have ice pop molds. You can still make these using small cups and ice pop sticks instead. To keep the sticks in place while freezing, arrange the cups on a tray and place the sticks in the smoothies. Cover with a piece of aluminum foil, poking holes in it where the sticks stand to hold them upright until frozen.

PER SERVING: Calories: 70; Total Fat: 2g; Protein: 5g; Carbohydrates: 9g; Sugars: 2g; Fiber: 3g; Sodium: 28mg

Grilled Peach and Coconut Yogurt Bowls

Gluten-Free | Vegetarian | 5-Ingredient | 30 Minutes or Less

Sometimes when looking for things to satisfy our sweet tooth, we overlook nature's original dessert: fruit. Grilling the peaches caramelizes some of their naturally occurring sugars and makes it so easy to turn ordinary pieces of stone fruit into a dessert masterpiece. Coconut and pistachios add a little extra sweetness and depth to this simple dessert.

CARBS PER SERVING: 11g

SERVINGS: 4 (½ peach each)

PREP TIME: 5 minutes

COOK TIME: 10 minutes

2 peaches, halved and pitted

½ cup plain nonfat Greek yogurt

1 teaspoon pure vanilla extract

¼ cup unsweetened dried coconut flakes

2 tablespoons unsalted pistachios, shelled and broken into pieces

1. Preheat the broiler to high. Arrange the rack in the closest position to the broiler.

2. In a shallow pan, arrange the peach halves, cut-side up. Broil for 6 to 8 minutes until browned, tender, and hot.

3. In a small bowl, mix the yogurt and vanilla.

4. Spoon the yogurt into the cavity of each peach half.

5. Sprinkle 1 tablespoon of coconut flakes and 1½ teaspoons of pistachios over each peach half. Serve warm.

Substitution tip: Use other stone fruit in place of peaches, as available. Nectarines, plums, and fresh apricots make great alternatives.

PER SERVING: Calories: 102; Total Fat: 5g; Protein: 5g; Carbohydrates: 11g; Sugars: 8g; Fiber: 2g; Sodium: 12mg

Chocolate Peanut Butter Freezer Bites

Gluten-Free | Vegetarian | Dairy-Free | No-Cook | 5-Ingredient | 30 Minutes or Less

If you love chocolate, you are going to love these little bites. Using just four basic ingredients, these are super easy to pull together and are a satisfying snack when your sweet tooth hits. Store them in the freezer and they'll last for over a month, giving you plenty to have on hand when you need a little boost of energy.

CARBS PER SERVING: 3g
SERVINGS: 32 (1 bite each)
PREP TIME: 5 minutes

1 cup coconut oil, melted

¼ cup cocoa powder

¼ cup honey

¼ cup natural peanut butter

1. Pour the melted coconut oil into a medium bowl. Whisk in the cocoa powder, honey, and peanut butter.

2. Transfer the mixture to ice cube trays in portions about 1½ teaspoons each.

3. Freeze for 2 hours or until ready to serve.

Technique tip: If you don't have enough ice cube trays on hand, you can also spread the mixture onto a parchment paper–lined baking sheet and freeze for about 30 minutes until set. Cut into squares and store frozen in an airtight container until you're ready to serve.

PER SERVING: Calories: 80; Total Fat: 8g; Protein: 1g; Carbohydrates: 3g; Sugars: 2g; Fiber: 0g; Sodium: 20mg

Dark Chocolate Almond Butter Cups

Gluten-Free | Vegan | Dairy-Free | No-Cook | 5-Ingredient

You are about to look at your muffin tins in a whole new way. These easy dessert cups can be made with four simple ingredients and are the perfect treat to grab when you are looking to satisfy your sweet tooth. Keep them in the freezer so you have one when desired. And with only 6 grams of carbs per cup, you can enjoy them often.

CARBS PER SERVING: 6g
SERVINGS: 12
PREP TIME: 15 minutes, plus 40 minutes for freezing

½ cup natural almond butter

1 tablespoon pure maple syrup

1 cup dark chocolate chips

1 tablespoon coconut oil

1. Line a 12-cup muffin tin with cupcake liners.

2. In a medium bowl, mix the almond butter and maple syrup. If necessary, heat in the microwave to soften slightly.

3. Spoon about 2 teaspoons of the almond butter mixture into each muffin cup and press down to fill.

4. In a double boiler or the microwave, melt the chocolate chips. Stir in the coconut oil, and mix well to incorporate.

5. Drop 1 tablespoon of chocolate on top of each almond butter cup.

6. Freeze for at least 30 minutes to set. Thaw for 10 minutes before serving.

Substitution tip: No almond butter? No problem. Use natural peanut butter instead.

PER SERVING: Calories: 101; Total Fat: 8g; Protein: 3g; Carbohydrates: 6g; Sugars: 4g; Fiber: 1g; Sodium: 32mg

Carrot Cake Bites

Gluten-Free | Vegan | Dairy-Free | No-Cook | 30 Minutes or Less

I've always preferred carrot cake to any other type of cake. In fact, one of the layers of our wedding cake was carrot, if you can believe it! So rest assured these bites are fellow-carrot-cake-lover approved and full of all the flavor from the traditional cake, minus some of the unwanted sugar.

CARBS PER SERVING: 10g
SERVINGS: 20 (1 bite each)
PREP TIME: 15 minutes

½ cup old-fashioned oats

2 medium carrots, chopped

6 dates, pitted

½ cup chopped walnuts

½ cup coconut flour

2 tablespoons hemp seeds

2 teaspoons pure maple syrup

1 teaspoon ground cinnamon

½ teaspoon ground nutmeg

1. In a blender jar, combine the oats and carrots, and process until finely ground. Transfer to a bowl.

2. Add the dates and walnuts to the blender and process until coarsely chopped. Return the oat-carrot mixture to the blender and add the coconut flour, hemp seeds, maple syrup, cinnamon, and nutmeg. Process until well mixed.

3. Using your hands, shape the dough into balls about the size of a tablespoon.

4. Store in the refrigerator in an airtight container for up to 1 week.

Option tip: These cake bites are great on their own, or you can top them for even more fun. Roll the finished balls in coconut flakes or unsweetened cocoa powder for a unique twist, or melt some white or dark chocolate and drizzle it on the balls before refrigerating.

PER SERVING: Calories: 68; Total Fat: 3g; Protein: 2g; Carbohydrates: 10g; Sugars: 6g; Fiber: 2g; Sodium: 6mg

Strawberry Cream Cheese Crepes

Gluten-Free | Vegetarian | 30 Minutes or Less

One of the best perks of living in California is the fresh local produce available year-round. Our favorite farmers' market find is strawberries; you just can't beat a ripe strawberry! You may not realize that strawberries are an amazing source of vitamin C, with just 8 strawberries providing more than 100 percent of your daily vitamin C needs. And since strawberries are one of the best diabetes-friendly, low-glycemic fruits, they are the perfect addition to these crepes.

CARBS PER SERVING: 20g
SERVINGS: 4 (1 crepe each)
PREP TIME: 10 minutes
COOK TIME: 10 minutes

½ cup old-fashioned oats

1 cup unsweetened plain almond milk

1 egg

3 teaspoons honey, divided

Nonstick cooking spray

2 ounces low-fat cream cheese

¼ cup low-fat cottage cheese

2 cups sliced strawberries

1. In a blender jar, process the oats until they resemble flour. Add the almond milk, egg, and 1½ teaspoons honey, and process until smooth.

2. Heat a large skillet over medium heat. Spray with nonstick cooking spray to coat.

3. Add ¼ cup of oat batter to the pan and quickly swirl around to coat the bottom of the pan and let cook for 2 to 3 minutes. When the edges begin to turn brown, flip the crepe with a spatula and cook until lightly browned and firm, about 1 minute. Transfer to a plate. Continue with the remaining batter, spraying the skillet with nonstick cooking spray before adding more batter. Set the cooked crepes aside, loosely covered with aluminum foil, while you make the filling.

4. Clean the blender jar, then combine the cream cheese, cottage cheese, and remaining 1½ teaspoons honey, and process until smooth.

5. Fill each crepe with 2 tablespoons of the cream cheese mixture, topped with ¼ cup of strawberries. Serve.

Substitution tip: Strawberries pair so well with the savory cream cheese filling, but other berries can work just as well. Substitute blueberries, blackberries, raspberries, or any other seasonal berries for great results.

PER SERVING: Calories: 149; Total Fat: 6g; Protein: 6g; Carbohydrates: 20g; Sugars: 10g; Fiber: 3g; Sodium: 177mg

Cream Cheese Swirl Brownies

Gluten-Free | Vegetarian | Nut-Free | 30 Minutes or Less

Brownies are the ultimate crowd-pleaser, and I wanted to make sure to add a brownie recipe to this cookbook to assure you that your favorite foods can continue to be your favorite foods. No food is always off-limits when it comes to managing your blood sugar levels, and brownies are (thankfully!) no exception. I hope you enjoy these brownies, savoring every bite, knowing that they are diabetes-friendly and good enough for the entire family.

CARBS PER SERVING: 6g

SERVINGS: 12

(1 brownie each)

PREP TIME: 10 minutes

COOK TIME: 20 minutes

2 eggs

¼ cup unsweetened applesauce

¼ cup coconut oil, melted

3 tablespoons pure maple syrup, divided

¼ cup unsweetened cocoa powder

¼ cup coconut flour

¼ teaspoon salt

1 teaspoon baking powder

2 tablespoons low-fat cream cheese

1. Preheat the oven to 350°F. Grease an 8-by-8-inch baking dish.

2. In a large mixing bowl, beat the eggs with the applesauce, coconut oil, and 2 tablespoons of maple syrup.

3. Stir in the cocoa powder and coconut flour, and mix well. Sprinkle the salt and baking powder evenly over the surface and mix well to incorporate. Transfer the mixture to the prepared baking dish.

4. In a small, microwave-safe bowl, microwave the cream cheese for 10 to 20 seconds until softened. Add the remaining 1 tablespoon of maple syrup and mix to combine.

5. Drop the cream cheese onto the batter, and use a toothpick or chopstick to swirl it on the surface. Bake for 20 minutes, until a toothpick inserted in the center comes out clean. Cool and cut into 12 squares.

6. Store refrigerated in a covered container for up to 5 days.

Option tip: Sprinkle ½ cup of chopped walnuts on the top before baking to make a heartier treat.

PER SERVING: Calories: 84; Total Fat: 6g; Protein: 2g; Carbohydrates: 6g; Sugars: 4g; Fiber: 2g; Sodium: 93mg

Oatmeal Cookies

Gluten-Free | Vegetarian | Dairy-Free | 30 Minutes or Less

We all need to indulge in a sweet treat every now and then, and warm oatmeal cookies are one of my favorites! Remember that having diabetes does not mean you can't eat dessert, and this recipe will show you it's more than possible to enjoy sweets *and* well-controlled blood sugar levels. This cookie has reduced carbs and sugar while still providing nutritious ingredients. I love making these for my toddler son, and I hope you will enjoy baking them for your family and friends as well!

CARBS PER SERVING: 5g
SERVINGS: 16
(1 cookie each)
PREP TIME: 5 minutes
COOK TIME: 15 minutes

¾ cup almond flour

¾ cup old-fashioned oats

¼ cup shredded unsweetened coconut

1 teaspoon baking powder

1 teaspoon ground cinnamon

¼ teaspoon salt

¼ cup unsweetened applesauce

1 large egg

1 tablespoon pure maple syrup

2 tablespoons coconut oil, melted

1. Preheat the oven to 350°F.

2. In a medium mixing bowl, combine the almond flour, oats, coconut, baking powder, cinnamon, and salt, and mix well.

3. In another medium bowl, combine the applesauce, egg, maple syrup, and coconut oil, and mix. Stir the wet mixture into the dry mixture.

4. Form the dough into balls a little bigger than a tablespoon and place on a baking sheet, leaving at least 1 inch between them. Bake for 12 minutes until the cookies are just browned. Remove from the oven and let cool for 5 minutes.

5. Using a spatula, remove the cookies and cool on a rack.

Technique tip: To keep your cookies from spreading too much in the oven, chill the dough for 30 minutes in the refrigerator before baking. The coconut oil will firm up, and you will end up with a thicker cookie.

PER SERVING: Calories: 76; Total Fat: 6g; Protein: 2g; Carbohydrates: 5g; Sugars: 1g; Fiber: 1g; Sodium: 57mg

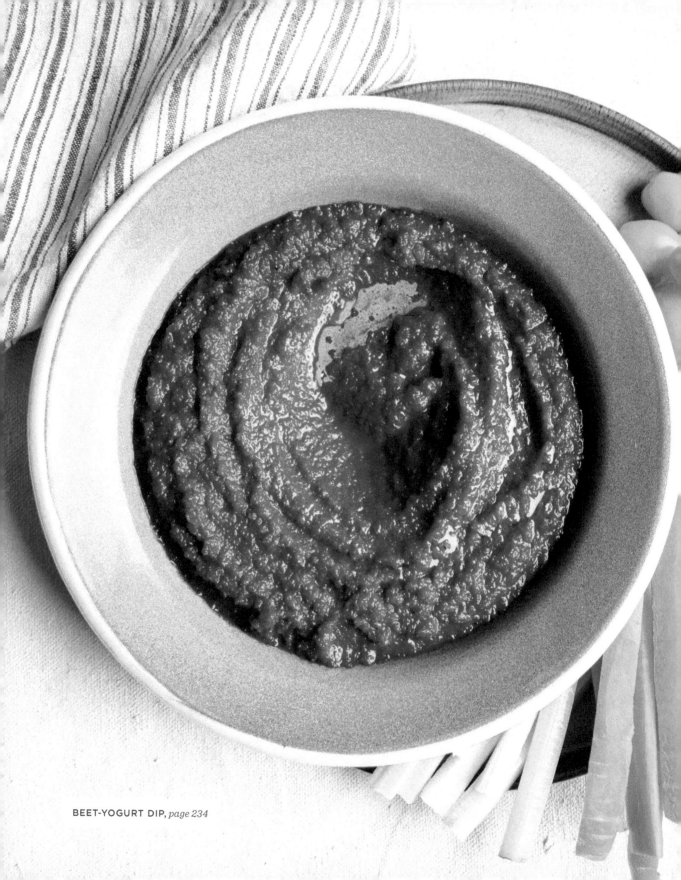

BEET-YOGURT DIP, *page 234*

14

Sauces, Dips, and Dressings

Low-Carb No-Cook Tomato Ketchup

Gluten-Free | Vegetarian | Dairy-Free | Nut-Free | No-Cook | 30 Minutes or Less

When you start looking at labels, one that can be particularly concerning is ketchup. Most brands contain a lot of added sugar. The good news is that you can make ketchup at home in little time and have a condiment you can feel good about eating that tastes great, too!

CARBS PER SERVING: 6g

SERVINGS: 32

(2 tablespoons each)

PREP TIME: 10 minutes

1 (28-ounce) can whole tomatoes, drained

2 (6-ounce) cans tomato paste

1 tablespoon olive oil

2 garlic cloves, peeled

⅓ cup apple cider vinegar

1 tablespoon dried minced onion

½ teaspoon ground cloves

1 teaspoon salt

¼ cup honey

1. In a blender jar, combine the tomatoes, tomato paste, olive oil, garlic, vinegar, onion, cloves, salt, and honey. Process until smooth. Taste and adjust the spices and seasonings as needed.

2. Transfer to airtight storage jars, cover tightly, and refrigerate for up to 3 weeks.

Option tip: This ketchup is not going to taste as sweet as store-bought varieties, but the true tomato flavor shines through in a big way. If you think it needs a little more sweetness, add a small amount more honey and adjust the flavors to your taste. Each time you make it, try to add a little less and see if you notice the difference.

PER SERVING: Calories: 29; Total Fat: 1g; Protein: 1g; Carbohydrates: 6g; Sugars: 5g; Fiber: 1g; Sodium: 104mg

Quick Tomato Marinara

Gluten-Free Vegan Dairy-Free Nut-Free 5-Ingredient 30 Minutes or Less

Marinara sauce makes an appearance in so many dishes, and commercial varieties are often loaded with sugar, salt, and other additives. This homemade variety is simple to make and so much better for you. The bonus is that it is more fresh tasting than most store-bought varieties. Using canned whole tomatoes imparts the most flavor and allows you to have this quick marinara ready in no time.

CARBS PER SERVING: 4g
SERVINGS: 8 (¼ cup each)
PREP TIME: 5 minutes
COOK TIME: 15 minutes

1 (28-ounce) can whole tomatoes

2 tablespoons extra-virgin olive oil

4 garlic cloves, minced

½ teaspoon salt

¼ teaspoon dried oregano

1. Discard about half of the liquid from the can of tomatoes, and transfer the tomatoes and remaining liquid to a large bowl. Use clean hands or a large spoon to break the tomatoes apart.

2. In a large skillet, heat the olive oil over medium heat. Add the garlic and salt, and cook until the garlic just begins to sizzle, without letting it brown.

3. Add the tomatoes and their liquid to the skillet.

4. Simmer the sauce for about 15 minutes until the oil begins to separate and become dark orange and the sauce thickens. Add the oregano, stir, and remove from the heat.

5. After the marinara has cooled to room temperature, store in glass containers in the refrigerator for up to 3 or 4 days, or in zip-top freezer bags for up to 4 months.

Option tip: **For a sauce with some kick, add ¼ teaspoon cayenne pepper along with the oregano.**

PER SERVING: Calories: 48; Total Fat: 4g; Protein: 1g; Carbohydrates: 4g; Sugars: 2g; Fiber: 1g; Sodium: 145mg

Fresh Tomato Salsa

Gluten-Free | Vegan | Dairy-Free | Nut-Free | No-Cook | 5-Ingredient | 30 Minutes or Less

Fresh salsa is one of the easiest ways to add more flavor to your food while also providing essential nutrients. Onions, tomatoes, and limes are all great sources of vitamin C, which helps promote healthy aging and prevents heart disease. Vitamin C is not heat stable, so for best absorption, you want to eat it raw—which is exactly how salsa is made. So go ahead and have double and triple servings of this salsa; there's no need to hold back.

CARBS PER SERVING: 4g
SERVINGS: 6 (¼ cup each)
PREP TIME: 10 minutes

2 or 3 medium, ripe tomatoes, diced

½ red onion, minced

1 serrano pepper, seeded and minced

Juice of 1 lime

¼ cup minced fresh cilantro

¼ teaspoon salt

1. In a small bowl, combine the tomatoes, onion, serrano pepper, lime juice, cilantro, and salt, and mix well. Taste and season with additional salt as needed.

2. Serve immediately, or transfer to an airtight container and refrigerate for up to 3 days.

Technique tip: When chopping chiles, use gloves or some other protection to prevent the oils from getting on your skin. Be sure to always wash your hands thoroughly after handling hot peppers, and avoid touching your eyes for several hours.

PER SERVING: Calories: 18; Total Fat: 0g; Protein: 1g; Carbohydrates: 4g; Sugars: 1g; Fiber: 1g; Sodium: 84mg

Quick Guacamole

Gluten-Free | Vegan | Dairy-Free | Nut-Free | No-Cook | 30 Minutes or Less

Traditional guacamole is not high in carbs, and this quick version is no different. When it comes to eating guac, it's all about what you pair it with. Think outside of the box about ways to eat guacamole. It can be used on salads, as a veggie dip, as a sauce on top of your favorite lean protein, and even as a spread on sandwiches.

CARBS PER SERVING: 6g

SERVINGS: 6 (¼ cup each)

PREP TIME: 10 minutes

2 large avocados

1 small, firm tomato, finely diced

¼ white onion, finely diced

¼ cup finely chopped fresh cilantro

2 tablespoons freshly squeezed lime juice

¼ teaspoon salt

Freshly ground black pepper

1. Cut the avocados in half, remove the seeds, and scoop out the flesh into a medium bowl.

2. Using a fork, mash the avocado flesh. Mix in the tomato, onion, cilantro, lime juice, and salt. Season with black pepper.

3. Serve immediately.

Technique tip: If you prefer a chunkier guacamole, go light on the mashing in step 2. The consistency of guacamole is all based on preference, so anywhere from a purée to chunky is fine, depending on how you like it.

PER SERVING: Calories: 82; Total Fat: 7g; Protein: 1g; Carbohydrates: 6g; Sugars: 1g; Fiber: 3g; Sodium: 84mg

Beet-Yogurt Dip

Gluten-Free | Vegetarian | Nut-Free

This bright and beautiful beet dip will definitely be the highlight at your next party or social gathering. Beets are incredibly nutritious and contain fiber, potassium, folate, and vitamin A. This translates to a delicious way to eat more vegetables and improve your health at the same time. With only 5 grams of carbs per serving, feel free to use this as a salad dressing or vegetable dip, or serve alongside your favorite lean protein.

CARBS PER SERVING: 5g
SERVINGS: 6 (¼ cup each)
PREP TIME: 10 minutes, plus 1 hour to chill
COOK TIME: 45 to 60 minutes

½ pound red beets

½ cup plain nonfat Greek yogurt

1 tablespoon extra-virgin olive oil

1 tablespoon freshly squeezed lemon juice

1 garlic clove, peeled

1 teaspoon minced fresh thyme

½ teaspoon onion powder

¼ teaspoon salt

1. Preheat the oven to 375°F.

2. Wrap the beets in aluminum foil and bake for 45 to 60 minutes until the beets are tender when pierced with a fork. Set aside and let cool for at least 10 minutes. Using your hands, remove the skins and transfer the beets to a blender.

3. To the blender jar, add the yogurt, olive oil, lemon juice, garlic, thyme, onion powder, and salt. Process until smooth. Chill for 1 hour before serving.

Make-ahead tip: Make this up to 3 days ahead and use for snacking throughout the week. It pairs well with crunchy vegetables like radishes, jicama, and celery.

PER SERVING: Calories: 49; Total Fat: 2g; Protein: 3g; Carbohydrates: 5g; Sugars: 3g; Fiber: 1g; Sodium: 121mg

Cucumber-Yogurt Dip

Gluten-Free | Vegetarian | Nut-Free | No-Cook | 5-Ingredient | 30 Minutes or Less

Whether using it as a dip or a spread, you will love the deliciously simple flavor of this yogurt-based staple. It works great with veggies, on falafel, or just spread on a piece of whole-grain pita. To use it as a dressing, add a little water to thin it out and pour away.

CARBS PER SERVING: 3g
SERVINGS: 6 (¼ cup each)
PREP TIME: 10 minutes

1 medium cucumber, peeled and grated

¼ teaspoon salt

1 cup plain nonfat Greek yogurt

2 garlic cloves, minced

1 tablespoon freshly squeezed lemon juice

1 tablespoon extra-virgin olive oil

¼ teaspoon freshly ground black pepper

1. In a colander, sprinkle the cucumber with the salt. Set aside.

2. In a medium bowl, combine the yogurt, garlic, lemon juice, olive oil, and pepper.

3. Using your hands, squeeze as much water from the grated cucumber as possible. Transfer the cucumber to the yogurt mixture and stir well. Cover and refrigerate for 2 hours, if desired, to let the flavors merge.

4. Store in the refrigerator in an airtight container for up to 5 to 7 days.

Option tip: If you like, add ½ teaspoon ground cumin to the dip for a little different flavor.

PER SERVING: Calories: 48; Total Fat: 3g; Protein: 4g; Carbohydrates: 3g; Sugars: 2g; Fiber: 0g; Sodium: 104mg

Caramelized Onion and Greek Yogurt Dip

Gluten-Free | Vegetarian | Nut-Free | 5-Ingredient

Onions have strong antioxidant, anti-inflammatory, antibiotic, and antiviral properties, but probably the most compelling reason to use them is their flavor. A perfect complement to virtually any savory dish, onions are even more amazing when caramelized. It takes a while to get them to the perfect golden state, so this is a good project to do when you are prepping food for the week or some other kitchen task nearby where you can keep watch but not have to be overly involved as the onions caramelize.

CARBS PER SERVING: 7g
SERVINGS: 8 (¼ cup each)
PREP TIME: 10 minutes
COOK TIME: 45 minutes

2 tablespoons extra-virgin olive oil

3 cups chopped onions

1 garlic clove, minced

2 cups plain nonfat Greek yogurt

1 teaspoon salt

Freshly ground black pepper

1. In a large pot, heat the olive oil over medium heat until shimmering. Add the onions, and stir well to coat. Reduce heat to low, cover, and cook for 45 minutes, stirring every the 5 to 10 minutes, until well-browned and caramelized. Add the garlic and stir until just fragrant.

2. Remove from the heat and let cool for 10 minutes.

3. In a mixing bowl, combine the onions, yogurt, salt, and pepper.

Make-ahead tip: Make this up to 3 days in advance, store in an airtight container in the refrigerator, and stir well before serving.

PER SERVING: Calories: 83; Total Fat: 4g; Protein: 6g; Carbohydrates: 7g; Sugars: 5g; Fiber: 1g; Sodium: 264mg

Miso-Ginger Dressing

Vegan | Dairy-Free | Nut-Free | No-Cook | 5-Ingredient | 30 Minutes or Less

Miso is a fermented paste made from soybeans, rice, and/or barley; koji (a fermenting agent); and salt. The salty condiment is a staple in Japanese cooking and a concentrated source of protein containing eight essential amino acids. This simple dressing combines the salty flavor of miso with salad favorites of vinegar and oil for a flavor that will enliven everything from a bed of greens to roasted vegetables.

CARBS PER SERVING: 1g

SERVINGS: 4

(1 tablespoon each)

PREP TIME: 10 minutes

1 tablespoon unseasoned rice vinegar

1 tablespoon red or white miso

1 teaspoon grated fresh ginger

1 garlic clove, minced

3 tablespoons extra-virgin olive oil

1. In a small bowl, combine the vinegar and miso into a paste. Add the ginger and garlic, and mix well. While whisking, drizzle in the olive oil.

2. Store in the refrigerator in an airtight container for up to 1 week.

Ingredient tip: Miso is commonly sold at Asian supermarkets as well as in the refrigerated section of many well-stocked traditional or natural grocers. Look for an unpasteurized and naturally fermented version. Yellow and beige-colored misos typically are the most mild flavored, while red and darker misos have a much stronger flavor.

PER SERVING: Calories: 99; Total Fat: 10g; Protein: 1g; Carbohydrates: 1g; Sugars: 0g; Fiber: 0g; Sodium: 169mg

Easy Italian Dressing

Gluten-Free | Vegetarian | Dairy-Free | Nut-Free | No-Cook | 30 Minutes or Less

Italian dressing is a perfect addition to any green salad, but that doesn't mean you have to stop there when it comes to using this easy kitchen staple. Use it to marinate meat or chicken, or add it to your favorite roasted veggie for a quick burst of flavor.

CARBS PER SERVING: 0g

SERVINGS: 12

(1 tablespoon each)

PREP TIME: 5 minutes

¼ cup red wine vinegar

½ cup extra-virgin olive oil

¼ teaspoon salt

¼ teaspoon freshly ground black pepper

1 teaspoon dried Italian seasoning

1 teaspoon Dijon mustard

1 garlic clove, minced

1. In a small jar, combine the vinegar, olive oil, salt, pepper, Italian seasoning, mustard, and garlic. Close with a tight-fitting lid and shake vigorously for 1 minute.

2. Refrigerate for up to 1 week.

Option tip: Add red pepper flakes to the dressing to turn up the heat, or add a pinch or more of grated Parmesan cheese to further enhance the flavor.

PER SERVING: Calories: 81; Total Fat: 9g; Protein: 0g; Carbohydrates: 0g; Sugars: 0g; Fiber: 0g; Sodium: 52mg

Ranch Vegetable Dip and Dressing

Gluten-Free | Vegetarian | Dairy-Free | No-Cook | 30 Minutes or Less

This easy veggie dip is not just for dipping veggies; it's loaded with them, too. Using a base of creamy cauliflower, this is a dairy-free ranch-style dressing that's perfect to use on green salads, on grain bowls, or as a dipping sauce to accompany your favorite protein.

CARBS PER SERVING: 2g

SERVINGS: 8

(2 tablespoons each)

PREP TIME: 10 minutes

2 cups frozen cauliflower, thawed

½ cup unsweetened plain almond milk

2 tablespoons extra-virgin olive oil

2 tablespoons apple cider vinegar

1 garlic clove, peeled

2 teaspoons finely chopped scallions, both white and green parts

2 teaspoons finely chopped fresh parsley

1 teaspoon finely chopped fresh dill

½ teaspoon Dijon mustard

½ teaspoon onion powder

½ teaspoon salt

¼ teaspoon freshly ground black pepper

1. In a blender jar, combine the cauliflower, almond milk, oil, vinegar, garlic, scallions, parsley, dill, mustard, onion powder, salt, and pepper. Process until very smooth.

2. Serve immediately, or transfer to a jar, cover tightly with a lid, and store in the refrigerator for up to 3 days.

Option tip: Play around with the seasoning as you like for a different flavor. Other add-ins that taste great in this creamy dressing include oregano, thyme, and shallots.

PER SERVING: Calories: 42; Total Fat: 4g; Protein: 1g; Carbohydrates: 2g; Sugars: 1g; Fiber: 1g; Sodium: 149mg

The Dirty Dozen and the Clean Fifteen™

A nonprofit environmental watchdog organization called Environmental Working Group (EWG) looks at data supplied by the US Department of Agriculture (USDA) and the Food and Drug Administration (FDA) about pesticide residues. Each year it compiles a list of the best and worst pesticide loads found in commercial crops. You can use these lists to decide which fruits and vegetables to buy organic to minimize your exposure to pesticides and which produce is considered safe enough to buy conventionally. This does not mean they are pesticide-free, though, so wash these fruits and vegetables thoroughly.

These lists change every year, so make sure you look up the most recent one before you fill your shopping cart. You'll find the most recent lists, as well as a guide to pesticides in produce, at EWG.org/FoodNews.

DIRTY DOZEN

Apples
Celery
Cherries
Cherry tomatoes
Cucumbers
Grapes
Nectarines
Peaches
Spinach

Strawberries
Sweet bell peppers
Tomatoes

In addition to the Dirty Dozen, the EWG added two types of produce contaminated with highly toxic organophosphate insecticides:

Kale/Collard greens
Hot peppers

CLEAN FIFTEEN

Asparagus
Avocados
Cabbage
Cantaloupe
Cauliflower
Eggplant
Grapefruit
Honeydew melon

Kiwis
Mangoes
Onions
Papayas
Pineapples
Sweet corn
Sweet peas (frozen)

Measurement Conversions

Volume Equivalents (Liquid)

US STANDARD	US STANDARD (OUNCES)	METRIC (APPROXIMATE)
2 tablespoons	1 fl. oz.	30 mL
¼ cup	2 fl. oz.	60 mL
½ cup	4 fl. oz.	120 mL
1 cup	8 fl. oz.	240 mL
1½ cups	12 fl. oz.	355 mL
2 cups or 1 pint	16 fl. oz.	475 mL
4 cups or 1 quart	32 fl. oz.	1 L
1 gallon	128 fl. oz.	4 L

Oven Temperatures

FAHRENHEIT	CELSIUS (APPROXIMATE)
250°F	120°C
300°F	150°C
325°F	165°C
350°F	180°C
375°F	190°C
400°F	200°C
425°F	220°C
450°F	230°C

Volume Equivalents (Dry)

US STANDARD	METRIC (APPROXIMATE)
⅛ teaspoon	0.5 mL
¼ teaspoon	1 mL
½ teaspoon	2 mL
¾ teaspoon	4 mL
1 teaspoon	5 mL
1 tablespoon	15 mL
¼ cup	59 mL
⅓ cup	79 mL
½ cup	118 mL
⅔ cup	156 mL
¾ cup	177 mL
1 cup	235 mL
2 cups or 1 pint	475 mL
3 cups	700 mL
4 cups or 1 quart	1 L

Weight Equivalents

US STANDARD	METRIC (APPROXIMATE)
½ ounce	15 g
1 ounce	30 g
2 ounces	60 g
4 ounces	115 g
8 ounces	225 g
12 ounces	340 g
16 ounces or 1 pound	455 g

Resources

PRODUCTS MENTIONED IN THE BOOK:

Ak-Mak crackers, akmakbakeries.com

Dave's Killer Bread, www.daveskillerbread.com

Ezekiel 4:9 tortillas and bread, www.foodforlife.com

Wasa crispbreads, www.wasa-usa.com

ONLINE RESOURCES FOR RELIABLE DIABETES AND NUTRITION INFORMATION:

Everyday Health, www.everydayhealth.com

For the Love of Diabetes, fortheloveofdiabetes.com

Harvard Health, www.health.harvard.edu

Healthline, www.healthline.com

Lori Zanini Nutrition, www.lorizanini.com

Type2Diabetes.com

RECOMMENDED ORGANIZATIONS:

Academy of Nutrition and Dietetics, www.eatright.org

American Association of Diabetes Educators, www.diabeteseducator.org

American Diabetes Association, diabetes.org

Diabetes Sisters, diabetessisters.org

National Institute of Diabetes and Digestive and Kidney Diseases, www.niddk.nih.gov

References

American Diabetes Association. "Lifestyle Management: Standards of Medical Care in Diabetes—2018." *Diabetes Care* 41, Supplement (January 2018): S38–S50. doi.org/10.2337 /dc18-S004.

American Diabetes Association. "What Does Blood Glucose Management Mean?" Accessed January 9, 2018. http://www.diabetes.org /living-with-diabetes/treatment-and-care /blood-glucose-control/tight-diabetes -control.html.

American Heart Association. "Causes of Heart Failure." Accessed February 22, 2018. http:// www.heart.org/HEARTORG/Conditions /HeartFailure/CausesAndRisksForHeartFailure /Causes-of-Heart-Failure_UCM_477643 _Article.jsp#.WpJigeg-dz9.

Boule, N. G., E. Haddad, G. P. Kenny, G. A. Wells, and R. J. Sigal. "Effects of Exercise on Glyce-mic Control and Body Mass in Type 2 Diabetes Mellitus: A Meta-analysis of Controlled Clinical Trials." *Journal of the American Medical Asso-ciation* 286, no. 10 (September 2001): 1218–27. doi:10.1001/jama.286.10.1218.

Centers for Disease Control and Prevention. "National Diabetes Statistics Report, 2017." Accessed January 5, 2018. http://www.diabetes .org/assets/pdfs/basics/cdc-statistics-report -2017.pdf.

Centers for Disease Control and Prevention. "Only 1 in 10 Adults Get Enough Fruits or Vegetables." November 16, 2017. https://www.cdc.gov/media/releases/2017 /p1116-fruit-vegetable-consumption.html.

Centers for Disease Control and Prevention. "Sodium Fact Sheet." Accessed March 9, 2018. https://www.cdc.gov/dhdsp/data_statistics /fact_sheets/fs_sodium.htm.

Centers for Disease Control and Prevention. "The Surprising Truth about Prediabetes." Accessed January 15, 2018. https://www.cdc .gov/features/diabetesprevention/.

Duyff, Roberta Larson. *American Dietetic Asso-ciation Complete Food and Nutrition Guide,* 4th ed. New York: Houghton Mifflin Harcourt, 2012.

Holt, Richard I. G., Mary de Groot, and Sherita Hill Golden. "Diabetes and Depression." Current Diabetes Reports 14, no. 6 (June 2014): 491.

Khandouzi, Nafiseh, Farzad Shidfar, Asadollah Rajab, Tayebeh Rahideh, Payam Hosseini, and Mohsen Mir Taheri. "The Effects of Gin-ger on Fasting Blood Sugar, Hemoglobin A1c, Apolipoprotein B, Apolipoprotein A-I and Malondialdehyde in Type 2 Diabetic Patients." *Iranian Journal of Pharmaceutical Research* 14, no. 1 (winter 2015): 131–40. doi:10.5812 /ijem.57927.

Larsson, S. C., and A. Wolk. "Magnesium Intake and Risk of Type 2 Diabetes: A Meta-analysis." *Journal of Internal Medicine* 262, no. 2 (August 2007): 208–14. doi:10.1111/j.1365-2796.2007.01840.x.

Martin, Teresa, and R. Keith Campbell. "Vitamin D and Diabetes." *Diabetes Spectrum* 24, no. 2 (May 2011): 113–18. doi.org/10.2337/diaspect.24.2.113.

McMacken, M., and S. Shah. "A Plant-Based Diet for the Prevention and Treatment of Type 2 Diabetes." *Journal of Geriatric Cardiology* 14, no. 5 (May 2017): 342–54. doi:10.11909/j.issn.1671-5411.2017.05.009.

National Institutes of Health. "Magnesium Fact Sheet for Health Professionals." Accessed January 9, 2018. https://ods.od.nih.gov/factsheets/Magnesium-HealthProfessional/.

National Institutes of Health. "Vitamin D Fact Sheet for Health Professionals." Accessed January 9, 2018. https://ods.od.nih.gov/factsheets/VitaminD-HealthProfessional/.

Shukla, Alpana P., Radu G. Iliescu, Catherine E. Thomas, and Louis J. Aronne. "Food Order Has a Significant Impact on Postprandial Glucose and Insulin Levels." *Diabetes Care* 38, no. 7 (July 2015): e98–e99. doi.org/10.2337/dc15-0429.

Siri-Tarino, P. W., Q. Sun, F. B. Hu, and R. M. Krauss. "Meta-analysis of Prospective Cohort Studies Evaluating the Association of Saturated Fat with Cardiovascular Disease." *American Journal of Clinical Nutrition* 91, no. 3 (March 2010): 535–46. doi:10.3945/ajcn.2009.27725.

Taylor, Roy. "Type 2 Diabetes: Etiology and Reversibility." *Diabetes Care* 36, no. 4 (April 2013): 1047–55. doi.org/10.2337/dc12-1805.

Turner, R. C., C. A. Cull, V. Frighi, and R. R. Holman. "Glycemic Control with Diet, Sulfonylurea, Metformin, or Insulin in Patients with Type 2 Diabetes Mellitus: Progressive Requirement for Multiple Therapies (UKPDS 49). UK Prospective Diabetes Study (UKPDS) Group." *Journal of the American Medical Association* 281, no. 21 (June 1999): 2005–2012.

U.S. Department of Agriculture. "2015–2020 Dietary Guidelines: Answers to Your Questions." Updated January 7, 2016. https://www.choosemyplate.gov/2015-2020-dietary-guidelines-answers-your-questions.

U.S. Department of Agriculture. "Food Composition Databases." Accessed March 9, 2018. https://ndb.nal.usda.gov/ndb/.

Virtanen, J. K., J. Mursu, H. E. Virtanen, M. Fogelholm, J. T. Salonen, T. T. Koskinen, S. Voutilainen, and T. P. Tuomainen. "Associations of Egg and Cholesterol Intakes with Carotid Intima-media Thickness and Risk of Incident Coronary Artery Disease according to Apolipoprotein E Phenotype in Men: The Kuopio Ischaemic Heart Disease Risk Factor Study." *American Journal of Clinical Nutrition* 103, no. 3 (March 2016): 895–901. doi:10.3945/ajcn.115.122317.

Yang, Quanhe, Zefeng Zhang, Edward W. Gregg, W. Dana Flanders, Robert Merritt, and Frank B. Hu. "Added Sugar Intake and Cardiovascular Diseases Mortality among US Adults." *JAMA Internal Medicine* 174, no. 4 (April 2014): 516–24. doi:10.1001/jamainternmed.2013.13563.

INDEX

Acknowledgments

This book has been a beautiful culmination of expert insight, hard work,
an amazing team effort, and so much love!

Thanks to my team, who helped me get this book from idea to creation: Meg, Kim, Katherine, Joanna, and the entire staff at Callisto. I have felt so wonderfully supported throughout this process and, because of this, have been able to focus on the people I strive to help. Thank you so much for this!

To my many friends and family members who graciously tested so many recipes, I so appreciate your willingness, your time, and your wonderful honesty. Special thanks to the Roffles, Callinans, Buehlers, Olssons, Vosses, Kathy, Pili, Festa, David, Kelli (and baby Walker!), Mom, Dad, Gary, and Joyce.

Thank you to all the colleagues and friends who provided their expert review to make sure this book checked every box: Alissa Rumsey, Lindsey Stenovek, Carolyn Testa, Lisa Cimperman, and Marina Chaparro.

And to my amazing husband and business partner, Grant, whose support and love always keeps me going. And to our wonderful son, Preston, whose happy and (very!) energetic personality makes it all worth it!

Finally, to each and every person with diabetes who does the hard work to take control of your blood sugar every day, thank you for allowing me to be a small part of your journey and for the inspiration you continuously provide me.

About the Author

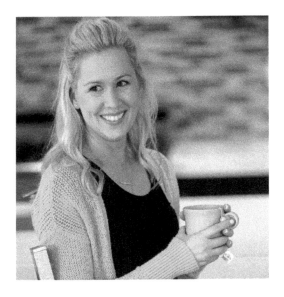

LORI ZANINI, RD, CDE, is a nationally recognized, award-winning food and nutrition expert. As a registered dietitian and certified diabetes educator,
she helps others learn how to lower their blood sugar without sacrificing
their lifestyle.

Lori earned a bachelor's degree in dietetics from Lipscomb University in her hometown of Nashville, Tennessee, and went on to complete her dietetic internship at Meredith College in Raleigh, North Carolina, where she was clinically trained at Duke University Hospital.

She is the co-creator of the online diabetes management program For the Love of Diabetes (ForTheLoveOfDiabetes.com), a proven and practical way
to reverse prediabetes and control type 2 diabetes.

She is the author of *Eat What You Love Diabetes Cookbook* and is featured regularly in both local and national media, including CNN, DoctorOz.com, Healthline, Everyday Health, SELF, Forbes, ABC7, and many others. She is a former national media spokesperson for the Academy of Nutrition and Dietetics.

Lori lives in Los Angeles, California, with her husband and son, where they try to stay caffeinated and as close to the beach as possible.

CONNECT WITH LORI ON SOCIAL MEDIA:

Facebook: @LoriZaniniNutrition
Instagram: @LoriZaniniNutrition
Twitter: @LoriTheRD